T0231147

LIVING THERAPY SERIES

Counselling for Obesity

Person-Centred Dialogues

Richard Bryant-Jefferies

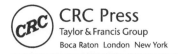

CRC Press
Taylor & Francis Group
Boca Raton London New York

CRC Press is an imprint of the
Taylor & Francis Group, an **informa** business

Radcliffe Publishing Ltd
18 Marcham Road
Abingdon
Oxon OX14 1AA
United Kingdom

www.radcliffe-oxford.com
Electronic catalogue and worldwide online ordering facility.

_____

© 2005 Richard Bryant-Jefferies

All rights reserved. No part of this publication may be reproduced, stored in a retrieval system or transmitted, in any form or by any means, electronic, mechanical, photo-copying, recording or otherwise, without the prior permission of the copyright owner.

British Library Cataloguing in Publication Data

A catalogue record for this book is available from the British Library.

ISBN 1 85775 758 9

Typeset by Aarontype Ltd, Easton, Bristol

Contents

Foreword

Tackling obesity is one of the biggest challenges of our time and one in which professionals struggle to provide treatments that will help individuals to fight against an obesogenic environment and move towards promoting healthier lifestyles and longevity of life. Government recommendations make pragmatic suggestions to 'eat less and exercise more'. If only it were that easy. Obesity is a complex multi-faceted disorder, which includes underlying psychological issues. It is my opinion that if the psychological aspects are not addressed, then once the 'intervention' is removed, be it a slimming club, medication or surgery, the eating problems will return and weight gain will be rapid. Perhaps this is why we have a thriving multi-billion pound slimming industry which prides itself on 1–5% success rates.

Radical changes in the treatment and management of obesity are required to promote permanent changes to both lifestyle and attitudes, and the psychology behind obesity needs to be urgently addressed before the epidemic gets out of hand. What a pleasure it was to read Richard's book. He succinctly highlights that the management of obesity is far more complex than symptom treatment, illustrating that we are merely managing the tip of the iceberg. What lies beneath are the deep psychological struggles which often govern individual eating patterns, as much with obesity as with any other eating disorder or disordered eating problem. Only when these issues are addressed can the process of weight loss begin.

Richard sensitively captures the complexities of the process of weight loss by using fictional case studies to illustrate the intricacy of obesity management from all dimensions, with an emphasis on psychological processing. The case studies are fascinating and the author has an exceptional ability to demonstrate a deep level of empathy with the clients he portrays, giving, in my experience, what I consider to be an accurate reflective insight into the psychological links to obesity, often related to personal life crisis and psychological trauma. His knowledge is well applied and, as well as offering insight into obesity as it affects women, he also offers a unique opportunity to gain a valuable insight into the world of men and obesity, both from the perceptive of the male therapist and the experiences of a male client.

As a therapist working in this field I found Richard's book provided me with questions which made me challenge my own practice and psychological approaches to working in this field. I am convinced that many professionals, and not only therapists, will find this book an invaluable resource for helping them to look beneath the surface of the symptoms of obesity and focus more on the contributing psychological factors. Only then can we say we will do our clients justice.

Kath Sharman
April 2005

Kath Sharman has a background in nursing, counselling, training, and child and adolescent health. She is now a consultant in obesity management and runs programmes called SHINE (Self Help, Independence, Nutrition and Exercise) for overweight children and adults.

Preface

In May 2004, the Health Committee of the House of Commons published its report on obesity. It makes stark reading.

> Should the gloomier scenarios relating to obesity turn out to be true, the sight of amputees will become much more familiar in the streets of Britain. There will be many more blind people. There will be huge demand for kidney dialysis. The positive trends of recent decades in combating heart disease, partly the consequence of the decline in smoking, will be reversed. Indeed, this will be the first generation where children die before their parents as a consequence of childhood obesity (House of Commons, 2004, p. 11).

The cause of obesity is not always simply the result of over-eating. There are also those for whom there is a genetic factor affecting their metabolism to induce extra weight. I wish to acknowledge this at the outset, however, this book focuses on obesity that follows on from excessive eating. The reasons why people over-eat, or eat foods that contribute to weight gain, are many and will vary from individual to individual. Over-eating *per se* is not necessarily a deliberate or conscious choice. As well as psychological reasons, or motivations related to body image, there will also be many people whose obesity is more the result of a lack of education or awareness of the effects of particular diets and lifestyles, and this may become linked to denial of the problem.

The reality is that obesity arises where there is an imbalance between the energy taken into the body through food, and the energy given out through maintaining the body and through exercise. The greater the imbalance, the greater the likelihood that obesity will develop.

All the books in the *Living Therapy* series (Radcliffe Publishing) aim to offer the reader an opportunity to experience and to appreciate, through the use of dialogue, some of the diverse and challenging issues that can arise during counselling. The success of the preceding books in the *Living Therapy* series, and the continued appreciative comments received from readers and by independent reviewers, is encouragement enough to once again extend this style into exploring the application of the person-centred approach to counselling and psychotherapy to another key area of difficulty within the human experience. Again and again people remark on how readable these books are and how much they bring the therapeutic process alive. In particular, students of counselling and psychotherapy have remarked on how accessible the text is. Trainers and others who are experienced in the field have indicated to me the timeliness of a series that focuses the application of the person-centred approach to working therapeutically with clients having particular issues. This is both heartening and encouraging. I want the style to draw people into the narrative and feel engaged with the characters and the therapeutic process. I want this series to be what I would term 'an experiential read'.

As with the other books in the *Living Therapy* series, *Counselling for Obesity: person-centred dialogues* is composed of fictitious dialogues between clients and their counsellors, and between the counsellors and their supervisors. Within the dialogues are woven the reflective thoughts and feelings of the clients, the counsellors and the supervisors, along with boxed comments on the process and references to person-centred theory. I do not seek to provide all the answers, or a technical manual expounding on the right way to work with clients who are experiencing an eating, or eating-related, issue. Rather I want to convey something of the process of working with representative material that can arise so that the reader may be stimulated into processing their own reactions, and reflecting on the relevance and effectiveness of the therapeutic responses, to thereby gain insight into themselves and their practice. Often it will simply lead to more questions which I hope will prove stimulating to the reader and encourage them to think through their own theoretical, philosophical and ethical positions and their boundary of competence.

Counselling for Obesity: person-centred dialogues is intended as much for experienced counsellors as it is for trainees and those new to counselling. It provides real insight into what can occur during counselling sessions. I hope it will raise awareness of, and inform, not only person-centred practice within this context, but also contribute to other theoretical approaches within the world of counselling, psychotherapy, and the various branches of psychology. Reflections on the therapeutic process and points for discussion are included to stimulate further thought and debate. Included in this book is material to inform the training process of counsellors and others who seek to work with issues of obesity and other eating disorders.

So, how does the person-centred counsellor approach working with a client who is experiencing the effects of over-eating or an eating issue that has generated a condition of obesity? I hope that this book will demonstrate the value, relevance and effectiveness of this approach, providing, as it does, a very human response to what is a very human problem. I hope that I am able to address a range of themes that leave you, the reader, with much to reflect on and to take into your professional counselling work, whatever the setting.

Richard Bryant-Jefferies
April 2005

About the author

Richard Bryant-Jefferies qualified as a person-centred counsellor/therapist in 1994 and remains passionate about the application and effectiveness of this approach. Between early 1995 and mid-2003 Richard worked at a community drug and alcohol service in Surrey as an alcohol counsellor. Since 2003 he has worked for the Central and North West London Mental Health NHS Trust, managing substance misuse service within the Royal Borough of Kensington and Chelsea in London. He has experience of offering both counselling and supervision in NHS, GP and private settings, and has provided training through 'alcohol awareness and response' workshops. He also offers workshops based on the use of written dialogue as a contribution to continuing professional development and within training programmes. His website address is: www.bryant-jefferies. freeserve.co.uk

Richard had his first book on a counselling theme published in 2001, *Counselling the Person Beyond the Alcohol Problem* (Jessica Kingsley Publishers), providing theoretical yet practical insights into the application of the person-centred approach within the context of the 'cycle of change' model that has been widely adopted to describe the process of change in the field of addiction. Since then he has been writing for the *Living Therapy* series (Radcliffe Publishing), producing an on-going series of person-centred dialogues: *Problem Drinking, Time Limited Therapy in Primary Care, Counselling a Survivor of Child Sexual Abuse, Counselling a Recovering Drug User, Counselling Young People, Counselling for Progressive Disability, Relationship Counselling: sons and their mothers, Responding to a Serious Mental Health Problem, Person-Centred Counselling Supervision: personal and professional, Counselling for Eating Disorders in Men, Counselling Victims of Warfare, Workplace Counselling in the NHS* and *Counselling for Problem Gambling*. The aim of the series is to bring the reader a direct experience of the counselling process, an exposure to the thoughts and feelings of both client and counsellor as they encounter each other on the therapeutic journey, and an insight into the value and importance of supervision.

Richard is also writing his first novel, 'Dying to Live', a story of traumatic loss, alcohol use and the therapeutic and has also adapted one of his books as a stage or radio play, and plans to do the same to other books in the series if the first is successful. However, he is currently seeking an opportunity for it to be recorded or staged.

Richard is keen to bring the experience of the therapeutic process, from the standpoint and application of the person-centred approach, to a wider audience. He is convinced that the principles and attitudinal values of this approach and the emphasis it places on the therapeutic relationship are key to helping people create greater authenticity both in themselves and in their lives, leading to a fuller and more satisfying human experience. By writing fictional accounts to try and bring the therapeutic process alive, to help readers engage with the characters within the narrative – client, counsellor and supervisor – he hopes to take the reader on a journey into the counselling room. Whether we think of it as pulling back the curtains or opening a door, it is about enabling people to access what can and does occur within the therapeutic process.

Acknowledgements

I would like to thank Kath Sharman who specialises in working with clients with obesity problems. Her comments on the draft of this book were particularly helpful. I would also like to thank her for contributing a Foreword to this book.

I also wish to thank everyone at Radcliffe Publishing for their continued support for this series.

Introduction

Counselling for Obesity: person-centred dialogues aims to demonstrate the counsellor's application of the person-centred approach (PCA) which is a theoretical approach that, at its heart, has the power of the relational experience. It is this experience which I believe to be the core of effective therapy, contributing to the possibility of releasing the client to realise greater potential for authentic living. The approach is widely used by counsellors working in the UK today. In a membership survey in 2001 by the British Association for Counselling and Psychotherapy, 35.6 per cent of those responding claimed to work to the person-centred approach, whilst 25.4 per cent identified themselves as psychodynamic practitioners. However, whatever the approach, it seems to me that the relationship is the key factor in contributing to a successful outcome though this must remain a very subjective concept for who, other than the client, can really define what experience is to be taken as a measure of a successful outcome?

This introduction presents information on the scale of the obesity problem, the use of language in addressing the issue and ideas for controlling what is eaten. There is also an introductory overview of person-centred theory, together with a description of Rogers' ideas as to the stages of psychological change and the characteristics of change within the person (*see* Appendix 1 on page 167).

Appendix 2 contains a description of the 'cycle of change' model that was originally developed by Prochaska and DiClemente (1982) and which has since been revised and developed further as part of the process of developing a fuller understanding of the stages that people pass through when changing a particular behaviour. Whilst this is not a person-centred framework *per se*, it does offer an interesting overview of stages of change and what kind of areas a person might focus on during the different stages. Finally, Appendix 3 offers ideas for 'Controlling what is eaten', with reference to Gilbert (2000).

Obesity

Obesity in England has grown by almost 400 per cent over the course of the last 25 years. Today, about three-quarters of the adult population are now overweight or obese (around 22 per cent are now obese). England has witnessed the fastest growth in obesity in Europe and childhood obesity has tripled in 20 years.

These are figures taken from the *Health Committee's Report on Obesity* (House of Commons, 2004) which also notes that:

- the average person now walks 189 miles per year compared to 255 miles 20 years ago
- levels of cycling have fallen by over 80% in the last 50 years
- fewer than 1% of school journeys are now made by bicycle
- half the nation's children fail to achieve the Government's modest target of two hours activity per week.

At the same time, energy-dense foods, which are highly calorific without being correspondingly filling, are becoming increasingly available, transport systems are also contributing to making it easy for people to consume more calories than they need. The report (House of Commons, 2004, p. 5) highlights the many barriers to the establishing of healthier diets:

- in the absence of practical cookery lessons, children and young people are growing up without the skills to prepare healthy meals, compounding reliance on convenience foods, which are often high in energy density
- healthy-eating messages are drowned out by the large proportion of advertising given over to highly energy-dense foods
- other types of food promotion, as well as pricing also make buying unhealthy food more attractive and economical than healthy alternatives
- food labelling, a key tool to help consumers choose healthy foods, is frequently either confusing or absent.

The report explains that humans have evolved to be very good at recognising hunger, but very bad at recognising satiety. While in times of uncertain food availability this symmetry could help people survive famines, in today's environment, it is very conducive to weight gain.

These factors contribute to the amount of energy going into our bodies, there is then the factor of how much energy we expend, particularly through exercise. The report states:

- only just over a third of men and around a quarter of women achieve the Department of Health's target of 30 minutes of physical activity five times a week
- levels of walking and cycling have fallen drastically in recent decades, while the number of cars has doubled in 30 years
- children are also increasingly sedentary both in and out of school. A fifth of boys and girls undertake less than 30 minutes activity a day
- television viewing has doubled since the 1960s, while physical activity is being squeezed out of daily life by the relentless march of automation (House of Commons, 2004, p. 205).

The health risks associated with obesity are many and severe. They include: 'Type 2 diabetes, gallbladder disease, dyslipidaemia, insulin resistance, breathlessness, sleep apnoea, hypertension, osteoarthritis (knees), coronary heart disease, low back pain, hyperuricaemia and gout, impaired fertility, anaesthetic risk, fetal defects associated with maternal obesity, cancer (breast cancer in postmenopausal

women, endometrial cancer, colon cancer), polycystic ovary syndrome, repro-
ductive hormone abnormalities' (House of Commons, 2004, p. 19).

The difficulty is that many obese or overweight people simply do not see it as a
problem, they have not experienced these detrimental effects to their health.
Some will take time for symptoms to emerge, and when they do, damage has
already been done. The normality of being larger has become established within
the social consciousness. But, as we have already seen, the risks to health from
obesity are many and serious.

Many psychological problems result from obesity as well. The National
Audit Office (NAO) Report in 2001, *Tackling Obesity in England*, noted that
'Obese people ... are more likely to suffer from a number of psychological problems, including binge-eating, low self-image and confidence, and a sense of
isolation and humiliation arising from practical problems.' Links to clinical
depression and higher suicide rates among obese women have also been indicated. It has been estimated that one in 13 deaths in the EU are likely to be related
to excess weight and within that figure the UK's figure of 8.7 per cent of deaths
attributable to excess weight is the highest (Banegas *et al.*, 2003).

The need for greater awareness and increased service provision within healthcare for people with obesity problems is also highlighted in the Health Commis-
sion's *Obesity Report*: 'We were appalled to learn of the desperate inadequacy of
treatment and support services for obese children. Obesity is a serious medical
problem ... patients with more entrenched or complex problems need prompt
access to specialist medical care. Childhood obesity is a worrying and increasingly common subset of this illness, and children in particular need specialist
care. Yet specialist obesity services seem to be an almost entirely neglected area
of the NHS ...' (House of Commons, 2004, p. 94).

The report also stresses a more holistic response to the problem, recommending
that: 'in establishing primary care obesity clinics, PCTs [primary care trusts]
should fully explore the possibilities of using less traditional models of service
delivery, involving clinicians from across the professional spectrum, from nurses
to pharmacists to dieticians. The full range of interventions available to treat obesity includes diet, lifestyle, medical treatment and surgical treatment' (House of
Commons, 2004, p. 92). The report also commented on the need to draw from
the expertise from commercial slimming organisations.

In their contribution to the *Obesity Report*, TOAST (The Obesity Awareness &
Solutions Trust) argues that amongst some groups, obesity was comparable to
addictive habits such as smoking or alcohol dependence:

> For many types of obese [people] there is a strong link to the problems of those
> with a drink problem; many talk of sometimes feeling out of control around
> food ... All the alcohol treatment programmes we know of use some form of
> counselling within their treatment profile. They recognise that the alcohol is
> often used as a coping mechanism, to drown sorrows, for swallowing anger,
> blotting out the pain, to be part of the crowd. Many overeaters will recog-
> nise these behaviours and reasons for over-consuming. Alcohol treatment
> programmes help people to recognise why they have been over consuming and

to find other coping mechanisms, helping clients build belief in them (House of Commons, 2004, p. 109).

The report concluded that 'it is vital that advances in medical and surgical treatment of obesity should be supported by equivalent development of services to address the psychological and behavioural aspects of obesity. All those receiving treatment for obesity, whether in a primary or in secondary care setting, should have access to psychological support provided by an appropriate professional, whether this is a psychiatrist, psychologist, psychotherapist, counsellor, or family therapist' (House of Commons, 2004, pp. 109–10).

The *Health Survey for England 2003* (Department of Health, 2004) shows that 'in terms of desirable levels of body mass index (BMI), the proportion of men with a desirable BMI (over 20 to 25) decreased from 37.8% in 1993 to 28.8% in 2003, while the proportion of men categorised as obese (BMI over 30) increased from 13.2% in 1993 to 22.9% in 2003. The proportion of women with a desirable BMI (over 20 to 25) decreased from 44.3% in 1993 to 37.3% in 2003. The proportion of women categorised as obese (BMI over 30) increased from 16.4% in 1993 to 23.4% in 2003. To summarise, 22.9% of men and 23.5% of women have a BMI rating above 30; the benchmark for obesity'. In addition, since 1993 the number of women with a BMI of 40 (indicating extreme obesity) has nearly tripled, and for men it is now five times higher than a decade ago.

People tend to make changes or to seek help for a problem when it reaches a point at which it has become uncomfortable or unacceptable. The need for greater public awareness is clear with a strong and joined-up response to ensure that producers are taking responsibility for promoting healthy eating, and consumers are informed enough to ensure that their choice of foodstuffs and lifestyle reflects greater personal responsibility for their health. A particular concern is the finding that, in 'a survey of 300 British families, only 25% of parents with overweight children recognised that their children were overweight. No fathers identified their sons as overweight, even when they were, and, perhaps even more disturbingly, 33% of mothers and 57% of fathers described their children as "normal" when in fact they were obese' (House of Commons, 2004, p. 95).

The distinct possibility is now being voiced that, if serious changes are not made to diet and lifestyle, then future decades will see children dying of obesity-related illnesses before their parents die. This, perhaps, is the most stark reminder that obesity is a problem that *has* to be addressed. Obesity has been described as 'one of the most devastating of diseases' (Adams, 1993, p. 109).

Language of obesity

In many publications, obesity is included under the term 'eating disorder'. This term is well recognised and widely used, but does it have application to obesity? And who judges when an eating pattern becomes disordered? When is it different to a social norm? The junk food culture today is a social norm but is argued by many to be behind the rise in obesity, as are the high consumption levels of sugar. So from a social norm perspective, overeating may be seen as normal, or has been seen as normal but now is being seriously questioned. But when an eating pattern brings with it serious health problems is it then to be categorised as a 'disorder', an 'eating issue' or a 'condition of obesity'? Should we introduce the word 'problematic' into the vocabulary when we think of eating; talking instead of 'problematic eating' perhaps, rather than regarding it as an 'eating disorder' which could be regarded as pathologising a particular behaviour.

Why do people eat? People eat particular foods for different reasons: for the taste, for the pleasant feeling of fullness, to conform to social norms, habit, to access social experiences, to experiment with new culinary experiences, because you have to in order to stay alive, to create a body with a particular kind of appearance. All are quite reasonable, however, there comes a point at which any of these can lead to a person's food intake generating a condition of obesity and, therefore, problems.

Coming, as I do, from a background of working with problem drinkers I see a need for a similar language to identify those people who have difficulties in relation to their eating pattern. Does the phrase, 'problem eaters' seem reasonable, though? It is certainly descriptive in terms of wanting to capture the idea of an eating pattern that causes problems and obesity is such a problem. But, not everyone is comfortable with 'problem drinkers', so it is likely that similar reactions will occur to 'problem eaters'. It seems that there is a challenge to be overcome in our use of language. I personally don't want to start seeing a term such as 'foodaholic' or 'overeater' to take root in the mass consciousness, as such a term certainly could end up defining a person in such a way that their other human qualities and talents become lost sight of. When someone says 'alcoholic' the image that it conjures up is often extreme and can certainly contain prejudicial thinking, we do not want the same to happen for people who, for whatever reason, are experiencing an obese condition.

We have to be careful that our use of language does not limit our perception of people. I have written elsewhere of the difficulties that arise when a label is attached to a person – the label becomes dominant and the person is lost sight of. Hence my first book was entitled *Counselling the Person Beyond the Alcohol Problem*. Maybe this book should be thought of as counselling the person beyond their obesity. I say this because a person-centred counsellor will not be treating obesity *per se*, but working with the whole person, with whatever that person wants to bring into the counselling relationship. It is likely that significant psychological and emotional factors are present, making their lives uncomfortable. These may be as a result of their size, the cause of their putting on weight, or a mixture of both. Whatever the cause of the person's obesity, relational factors will play a part – relationship with others and with themselves.

Dialogue format

The reader who has not read other titles in the *Living Therapy* series may find it takes a while to adjust to the dialogue format in the main body of the book.

Many of the responses offered by the counsellors, John and Pamela, are reflections of what their respective clients, Steve and Julia, have said. This is not to be read as conveying a simple repetition of the clients' words. Rather, the counsellor seeks to voice empathic responses, often with a sense of 'checking out' that they are hearing accurately what the clients are saying. The client says something; the counsellor then conveys what they have heard, what they sense the client has sought to communicate to them, sometimes with the same words, sometimes with words that include a sense of what they feel is being communicated through the client's tone of voice, facial expression, or simply the relational atmosphere of the moment. The client is then enabled to confirm that she has been heard accurately, or correct the counsellor in her perception. The client may then explore more deeply what they have been saying or move on, in either case with a sense that they have been heard and warmly accepted. To draw this to the reader's attention, I have included some of the inner thoughts and feelings that are present within the individuals who form the narrative.

The sessions are a little compressed. It is also fair to say that different clients will take different periods of time before choosing to disclose particular issues, and will also take varying lengths of time in working with their own process. This book is not intended to in any way indicate the length of time that may be needed to work with the kinds of issues that are being addressed. The counsellor needs to be open and flexible to the needs of the client. For some clients, the process would take a lot longer. But there are also clients who are ready to talk about difficult experiences almost immediately – sometimes not feeling that they have much choice in the matter as their own organismic processes are already driving memories, feelings, thoughts and experiences to the surface and into daily awareness.

The issues brought to counselling in the book cover a number of areas, and more. The client (Steve) in the first part of the book is overweight. His doctor has told him he has high blood pressure. He is also experiencing breathlessness which, again, the doctor has indicated is linked to his weight. Steve is unsure if he really has a problem, although deep down he knows he has, he just doesn't want people telling him what to do. He is also sensitive about his size where he is feeling judged. His eating is largely habitual though it is linked to experiences in his early life.

The second client (Julia) is experiencing a compulsive need to eat to maintain her weight, size and shape. This has its roots in difficult childhood experiences that caused her to feel the need to make herself unattractive to the attentions of boys and of men. Now, as a young woman, her eating is instinctively habitual, satisfying a range of needs but now having a problematic effect on her health – back problems. These two scenarios do not encompass all possible causes of obesity, they simply highlight some of the emotional factors that can be associated for some people. Others will have developed an obese condition for different reasons, however, the response from the person-centred approach will be similar to that described in this book. Also, if the gender mix of the clients and counsellors had been different the responses may have been different, and the relationship between counsellor and client more or less easy, and the reader may wish to bear this in mind as they read the book, considering where there might have been a different dialogue had there been a different gender mix. All characters in this book are fictitious and are not intended to bear resemblance to any particular person or persons.

Supervision

The supervision sessions are included in this book to offer the reader insight into the nature of therapeutic supervision in the context of the counselling profession, a method of supervising that I term 'collaborative-review'. For many trainee counsellors, the use of supervision can be something of a mystery, and it is hoped that this book will go a long way to unravelling this. In the supervision sessions I seek to demonstrate the application of the supervisory relationship. My intention is to show how supervision of the counsellor is very much a part of the process of enabling a client to work through issues that relate to obesity.

Many professions do not recognise the need for some form of personal and process supervision, and often what is offered is line-management. However, counsellors are required to receive regular supervision in order to explore the dynamics of the relationship with the client, the impact of the work on the counsellor and on the client, to receive support, to encourage professional development of the counsellor and to provide an opportunity for an experienced co-professional to monitor the supervisee's work in relation to ethical standards and codes of practice. The supervision sessions are included because they are an integral part of the therapeutic process. It is also hoped that they will help readers from other professions to recognise the value of some form of supportive and collaborative supervision in order to help them become more authentically present with their own clients. Merry describes what he termed as 'collaborative inquiry' as a 'form of research or inquiry in which two people (the supervisor and the counsellor) collaborate or co-operate in an effort to understand what is going on within the counselling relationship and within the counsellor'. He emphasises how this 'moves the emphasis away from "doing things right or wrong" (which seems to be the case in some approaches to supervision) to "how is the counsellor being, and how is that way of being contributing to the development of the counselling relationship based on the core conditions"' (2002, p. 173). Elsewhere, Merry describes the relationship between person-centred supervision and congruence, indicating that 'a state of congruence ... is the necessary condition for the therapist to experience empathic understanding and unconditional positive regard' (2001, p. 183). Effective person-centred supervision provides a means through which congruence can be promoted within the therapist.

Tudor and Worrall (2004) have drawn together a number of theoretical and experiential strands from within and outside of the person-centred tradition in order to develop a theoretical position on the person-centred approach to supervision. In my view, this is a timely publication, defining the necessary factors for effective supervision within this way of working, and the respective responsibilities of both supervisor and supervisee in keeping with person-centred values and principles. They contrast person-centred working with other approaches to supervision and emphasise the importance of the therapeutic space as a place within which practitioners 'can dialogue freely between their personal philosophy and the philosophical assumptions which underlie their chosen theoretical orientation' (Tudor and Worrall, 2004, pp. 94–5). They affirm the values and attitudes of person-centred working (which I will describe later in this introduction) and explore their application to the supervisory relationship.

There are, of course, as many models of supervision as there are models of counselling. In this book the supervisor is seeking to apply the attitudinal qualities of the person-centred approach.

It is the norm for all professionals working in the healthcare and social care environment in this age of regulation to be formally accredited or registered and to work to their own professional organisation's code of ethics or practice. For instance, registered counselling practitioners with the British Association for Counselling and Psychotherapy are required to have regular supervision and continuing professional development to maintain registration. Whilst professions other than counsellors will gain much from this book in their work, it is essential that they follow the standards, safeguards and ethical codes of their own professional organisation, and are appropriately trained and supervised to work on the issues that arise.

The person-centred approach

The person-centred approach (PCA) was formulated by Carl Rogers and references are made to his ideas within the text of this book. However, it will be helpful for readers who are unfamiliar with this way of working to have an appreciation of its theoretical base. Rogers proposed that certain conditions, when present within a therapeutic relationship, would enable the client to develop towards what he termed 'fuller functionality'. Over a number of years he refined these ideas, which he defined as 'the necessary and sufficient conditions for constructive personality change'. These he described as follow.

1   Two persons are in psychological contact.
2   The first, the client, is in a state of incongruence, being vulnerable or anxious.
3   The second person, the therapist, is congruent or integrated in the relationship.
4   The therapist experiences unconditional positive regard for the client.
5   The therapist experiences an empathic understanding of the client's internal frame of reference and endeavours to communicate this experience to the client.
6   The communication to the client of the therapist's empathic understanding and unconditional positive regard is to a minimal degree achieved (Rogers, 1957, p. 96).

Contact

The first necessary and sufficient condition given for constructive personality change is that of 'two persons being in psychological contact'. However, although he later published this as simply 'contact' (Rogers, 1959) it is suggested (Wyatt and Sanders, 2002, p. 6) that this was actually written in 1953–4. They quote Rogers as defining contact in the following terms: 'Two persons are in psychological contact, or have the minimum essential relationship when each makes a perceived or subceived difference in the experiential field of the other' (Rogers, 1959, p. 207). A recent exploration of the nature of psychological contact from a person-centred perspective is given by Warner (2002).

There is much to reflect on when considering a definition of 'contact' or 'psychological contact'. Contact can be described as 'all or nothing', i.e. present, or not, or as a continuum with greater or lesser degrees of contact possible. It seems to me that it is both. That rather like the way that light may be regarded as either a particle or a wave, contact may be seen as a specific state of being, or as a process, depending upon what the perceiver is seeking to measure or observe. If I am trying to observe or measure whether there is contact, then my answer will be in terms of 'yes' or 'no'. If I am seeking to determine the degree to which contact exists, then the answer will be along a continuum. In other words, from the moment of minimal contact there is contact, but that contact can then extend as more aspects of the client become present within the therapeutic relationship which, itself, may at times reach moments of increasing depth.

Empathy

Rogers defined empathy as meaning 'entering the private perceptual world of the other ... being sensitive, moment by moment, to the changing felt meanings which flow in this other person ... It means sensing meanings of which he or she is scarcely aware, but not trying to uncover totally unconscious feelings' (Rogers, 1980, p. 142). It is a very delicate process, and it provides a foundation block for effective person-centred therapy. The counsellor's role is primarily to establish empathic rapport and communicate empathic understanding to the client. This latter point is vital. Empathic understanding only has therapeutic value where it is communicated to the client.

There is so much more to empathy than simply letting the client know what you understand from what they have communicated. It is also, and perhaps more significantly, the actual *process* of listening to a client, of attending – facial expression, body language, and presence – that is being offered and communicated and received *at the time that the client is speaking, at the time that the client is experiencing what is present for them*. It is, for the client, the knowing that, in the moment of an experience the counsellor is present and striving to be an understanding companion.

Unconditional positive regard

Within the therapeutic relationship the counsellor seeks to maintain an attitude of unconditional positive regard towards the client and all that they disclose. This is not 'agreeing with', it is simply warm acceptance of the fact that the client is being how they need or choose to be. Rogers wrote, 'when the therapist is experiencing a positive, acceptant attitude towards whatever the client *is* at that moment, therapeutic movement or change is more likely to occur (Rogers, 1980, p. 116). Mearns and Thorne suggest that 'unconditional positive regard is the label given to the fundamental attitude of the person-centred counsellor towards her client. The counsellor who holds this attitude deeply values the humanity of her client and is not deflected in that valuing by any particular client behaviours. The attitude manifests itself in the counsellor's consistent acceptance of and enduring warmth towards her client' (Mearns and Thorne, 1988, p. 59).

Bozarth and Wilkins assert that 'unconditional positive regard is the curative factor in person-centred therapy' (Bozarth, 1998; Bozarth and Wilkins, 2001, p. vii). Drawing these two statements together it might then be suggested that the unconditional positive regard experienced and conveyed by the counsellor, and received by the client, as an expression of the counsellor's valuing of their client's humanity, has a curative role in the therapeutic process. To this can be added that this may be the case more specifically for those individuals who have been affected by a lack of unconditional warmth and prizing in their lives.

Congruence

Last, but by no means least, is that state of being that Rogers referred to as congruence, but which has also been described in terms of 'realness', 'transparency', 'genuineness' and 'authenticity'. Indeed Rogers wrote that '... genuineness, realness or congruence ... this means that the therapist is openly being the feelings and attitudes that are flowing within at the moment ... the term transparent catches the flavour of this condition' (Rogers, 1980, p. 115). Putting this into the therapeutic setting, we can say that 'congruence is the state of being of the counsellor when her outward responses to her client consistently match the inner feelings and sensations which she has in relation to her client' (Mearns and Thorne, 1999. p. 84). Interestingly, Rogers makes the following comment in his interview with Richard Evans that with regard to the three conditions, 'first, and most important, is therapist congruence or genuineness ... one description of what it means to be congruent in a given moment is to be aware of what's going on in your experiencing at that moment, to be acceptant towards that experience, to be able to voice it if it's appropriate, and to express it in some behavioural way' (Evans, 1975).

I would suggest that any congruent expression by the counsellor of their feelings or reactions has to emerge through the process of being in therapeutic relationship with the client. Indeed, the condition indicates that the therapist is 'congruent or integrated into the relationship'. This indicates the significance of the relationship. Being congruent is a disciplined way of being and not an open-door to endless self-disclosure. Congruent expression is perhaps most appropriate and therapeutically valuable where it is informed by the existence of an empathic understanding of the client's inner world, and is offered in a climate of a genuine warm acceptance towards the client. Having said that, it is reasonable to suggest that, taking Rogers' comment quoted earlier of regarding congruence as 'most important' we might suggest that unless the therapist is congruent in themselves and in the relationship, then their empathy and unconditional positive regard would be at risk of not being authentic or genuine.

Another view, however, would be that it is in some way false to distinguish or rather seek to separate out the three 'core conditions', that they exist together as a whole, mutually dependent on each others' presence in order to ensure that therapeutic relationship is established.

Perception

There is also the sixth condition, of which Rogers wrote: 'the final condition . . . is that the client perceives, to a minimal degree, the acceptance and empathy which the therapist experiences for him. Unless some communication of these attitudes has been achieved, then such attitudes do not exist in the relationship as far as the client is concerned, and the therapeutic process could not, by our hypothesis, be initiated' (Rogers, 1957). It is interesting that Rogers uses the words 'minimal degree', suggesting that the client does not need to fully perceive the fullness of the empathy and unconditional positive regard present within, and communicated by, the counsellor. A glimpse accurately heard and empathically understood is enough to have positive, therapeutic effect although logically one might think that the more that is perceived, the greater the therapeutic impact. But if it is a matter of intensity and accuracy, then a client experiencing a vitally important fragment of their inner world being empathically understood may be more significant to them, and more therapeutically significant, than a great deal being heard less accurately and with a weaker sense of the therapist's understanding. The communication of the counsellor's empathy, congruence and unconditional positive regard, received by the client, creates the conditions for a process of constructive personality change.

Relationship is key

The PCA regards the relationship that counsellors have with their clients, and the attitude that they hold within that relationship, to be key factors. In my experience, many adult psychological difficulties develop out of life-experiences that involve problematic, conditional or abusive relational experiences. This can be centred in childhood or later in life, and in this book we focus on the development of eating patterns and other associated behaviours which, themselves, become problematic. What is significant is that the individual is left, through relationships that have a negative conditioning effect, with a distorted perception of themselves and their potential as a person. Patterns are established in early life, bringing their own particular problems, however they can be exacerbated by conditional and psychologically damaging experiences later in life, that in some cases will have a resonance to what has occurred in the past, exacerbating the effects still further.

An oppressive experience can impact on a child's confidence in themselves, leaving them anxious, uncertain and moving towards establishing patterns of thought, feeling and behaviour associated with the developing concept of themselves typified by 'I am weak and cannot expect to be treated any differently'; 'I just have to accept this attitude towards me, what can I do to change anything?'. These psychological conclusions may rest on patterns of thinking and feeling already established, perhaps the person was bullied at school (possibly due to being over-weight), or experienced rejection in the home (and may have eaten excessively to fill an emotional void). They may have had a lifetime of stress (and overeaten as a comforter), or it may be a relatively new experience, either way a manner of thinking may develop typified by 'it's normal to feel stressed, you just keep going, whatever it takes' – that is until the day arrives when the person is so overloaded that they breakdown under the pressure, and may then require a significant length of time in order to recover.

The result is a conditioned sense of self, and an associated eating pattern which has meaning to this experience may have become firmly established. The individual will then think, feel and act in ways that enable them to maintain their self-beliefs and meanings within their learned or adapted concept of self. This is then lived out, the person seeking to satisfy what they have come to believe about themselves: needing to care either because it has been normalised, or in order to prove to themselves and the world that they are a 'good' person. They will need to maintain this conditioned sense of self and the sense of satisfaction that this gives them when it is lived out because they have developed such a strong identity with it. A particular eating pattern can be one factor in maintaining a particular sense of self, or in creating a new one in order to escape from discomfort.

Conditions of worth

The term, 'conditions of worth', applies to the conditioning mentioned previously that is frequently present in childhood, and at other times in life, when a person experiences that their worth is conditional on their doing something, or behaving, in a certain way. This is usually to satisfy someone else's needs, and can be contrary to the client's own sense of what would be a satisfying experience. The values of others become a feature of the individual's structure of self. The person moves away from being true to themselves, learning instead to remain 'true' to their conditioned sense of worth. And this conditioned sense of worth may be linked to an eating pattern – having to eat a lot to satisfy a parental need for a child that is 'big and strong', or to fit with a parental over-eating pattern, or an unhealthy diet with high levels of food that will increase weight. Or it could be that the child eats not out of habit imposed on them, but from their own need to experience a certain satisfaction that comes from a full stomach, or from other psychological effects from the chemicals in certain food-stuffs.

This conditioned state of being in the client is challenged by the person-centred therapist by offering them unconditional positive regard and warm acceptance. Such a therapist, by genuinely offering these therapeutic attitudes, provides the client with an opportunity to be exposed to what may be a new experience or one that in the past they have dismissed, preferring to stay with that which matches and therefore reinforces their conditioned sense of worth and sense of self. It can challenge that person's need to eat to feel good in themselves, to fill an emotional void, to sustain whatever the conditioning is that they have internalised.

By offering someone a non-judgemental, warm and accepting, and authentic relationship – (perhaps a kind of 'therapeutic love'?) – that person can grow into a fresh sense of self in which their potential as a person can become more fulfilled. It enables them to liberate themselves from the constraints of patterns of conditioning. Such an experience fosters an opportunity for the client to rede-fine themselves as they experience the presence of the therapist's congruence, empathy and unconditional positive regard. This process can take time. Often the personality change that is required to sustain a shift away from what have been termed 'conditions of worth' may require a lengthy period of therapeutic work, bearing in mind that the person may be struggling to unravel a sense of self that has been developed, sustained and reinforced for many decades of life. Of course, where they have been established more recently in their lives then less time may be necessary.

Actualising tendency

A crucial feature or factor in this process of 'constructive personality change' is the presence of what Rogers termed 'the actualising tendency', a tendency towards fuller and more complete personhood with an associated greater fulfil-ment of their potentialities. The role of the person-centred counsellor is to provide the facilitative climate within which this tendency can work constructively. The 'therapist trusts the actualizing tendency of the client and truly believes that the client who experiences the freedom of a fostering psychological climate will resolve his or her own problems' (Bozarth, 1998, p. 4). This is fundamental to the application of the person-centred approach. Rogers (1986, p. 198) wrote: 'the person-centred approach is built on a basic trust in the person . . . [It] depends on the actualising tendency present in every living organism – the tendency to grow, to develop, to realise its full potential. This way of being trusts the construc-tive directional flow of the human being towards a more complex and complete development. It is this directional flow that we aim to release.'

For some people, or for people at certain stages, rather than producing a liber-ating experience, there will instead be a tendency to maintain the status quo, perhaps the fear of change, the uncertainty, or the implications of change are such that the person prefers to maintain the known, the certain. In a sense, there is a liberation from the imperative to change and grow which may bring temporary – and perhaps permanent – relief for the person. The actualising tendency may work through the part of the person that needs relief from change, enhancing its presence for the period of time that the person experiences a need to maintain this. The person-centred therapist will not try to move the person from this place or state. It is to be accepted, warmly and unconditionally. And, of course, sometimes in the moment of acceptance the person is enabled to question whether that really is how they want to be.

Configuration within self

It is of value to draw attention, at this point, to the notion of 'configurations within self'. Configurations within self (Mearns and Thorne, 2000) are discrete sets of thoughts, feelings and behaviours that develop through the experience of life. They emerge in response to a range of experiences including the process of introjection and the symbolisation of experiences, as well as in response to dissonant self-experience within the person's structure of self. They can also exist in what Mearns terms as 'growthful' and 'not for growth', configurations (Mearns and Thorne, 2000, pp. 114–6), each offering a focus for the actualising tendency, the former seeking an expansion into new areas of experience with all that that brings, the latter seeking to energise the status quo and to block change because of its potential for disrupting the current order within the structure of self. The actualising tendency may not always manifest through growth or developmental change. It can also manifest through periods of stabilisation and stability, or a wanting to get away from something. The self, then, is seen as a constellation of configurations with the individual moving between them and living through them in response to experience.

Mearns suggests that these 'parts' or 'configurations' interrelate 'like a family, with an individual variety of dynamics'. As within any 'system', change in one area will impact on the functioning of the system. He therefore comments that 'when the interrelationship of configurations changes, it is not that we are left with something entirely new: we have the same "parts" as before, but some which may have been subservient before are stronger, others which were judged adversely are accepted, some which were in self-negating conflict have come to respect each other, and overall the parts have achieved constructive integration with the energy release which arises from such fusion' (Mearns and Thorne, 1999, pp. 147–8). The growing acceptance of the configurations, their own fluidity and movement within the self-structure, the increased, open and more accurate communication between the parts, is, perhaps, another way of considering the integrating of the threads of experience to which Rogers refers.

In terms of these ideas, we can anticipate clients containing, within themselves, particular configurations with which certain eating patterns or behaviours linked to appearance and weight are associated. So, a configuration may have developed that associates eating with being big and strong to ward off bullying at school, or eating to gain weight to avoid attractiveness and so reduce the risk of repeated sexual abuse, or to simply put people off from making sexual advances. It may be a configuration that has developed out of experiences that have caused the generation of a sense of self wracked with low self-esteem and a 'don't care' attitude to one's health and physical shape. A dominant configuration may develop that contains the many thoughts, feelings and behaviours associated with a person's over-eating pattern, with this configuration assuming a psychological primacy which, in turn, means the associated eating behaviour then also takes a similar position in the person's life. Over-eating may then become a means of maintaining the person's sense of self and identity.

There may also be 'not for eating' configurations as well, or these may emerge through the process of working at weight loss. Understanding the configurational nature of ourselves enables us to understand why we are triggered into certain thoughts, feelings and behaviours, and how they group together, serving a particular experiential purpose for the person.

From this theoretical perspective we can argue that the person-centred counsellor's role is essentially facilitative. Creating the therapeutic climate of empathic understanding, unconditional positive regard and authenticity creates a relational climate which encourages the client to move into a more fluid state with more openness to their own experience and the discovery of a capacity towards a fuller actualising of their potential.

Relationship re-emphasised

In addressing these factors the therapeutic relationship is central. A therapeutic approach such as person-centred affirms that it is not what you do so much as *how you are* with your client that is therapeutically significant, and this 'how you are' has to be received by the client. Gaylin (2001, p. 103) highlights the importance of client perception. 'If clients believe that their therapist is working on their behalf – if they perceive caring and understanding – then therapy is likely to be successful. It is the condition of attachment and the perception of connection that have the power to release the faltered actualisation of the self.' He goes on to stress how 'we all need to feel connected, prized – loved', describing human beings as 'a species born into mutual interdependence', and that there 'can be no self outside the context of others. Loneliness is dehumanising and isolation anathema to the human condition. The relationship,' he suggests 'is what psychotherapy is all about.'

'Love' is an important word though not necessarily one often used to describe therapeutic relationship. Patterson, however, gives a valuable definition of love as it applies to the person-centred therapeutic process. He writes, 'we define love as an attitude that is expressed through empathic understanding, respect and compassion, acceptance, and therapeutic genuineness, or honesty and openness towards others' (Patterson, 2000, p. 315). We all need love, but most of all we need it during our developmental period of life. The same author affirms that 'whilst love is important throughout life for the well-being of the individual, it is particularly important, indeed absolutely necessary, for the survival of the infant and for providing the basis for the normal psychological development of the individual' (Patterson, 2000, pp. 314–5).

In a previous book in this series I used the analogy of treating a wilting plant (Bryant-Jefferies, 2003b, p. 12). We can spray it with some specific herbicide or pesticide to eradicate a perceived disease that may be present in that plant, and that may be enough. But perhaps the true cause of the disease is that the plant is located in harsh surroundings, perhaps too much sun and not enough water, poor soil, near other plants that it finds difficulty in surviving so close to. Maybe by offering the plant a healthier environment that will facilitate greater nourishment according to the needs of the plant, it may become the strong, healthy plant it has the potential to become. Yes, the chemical intervention may also be helpful, but if the true causes of the diseases are environmental – essentially the plant's relationship with that which surrounds it – then it won't actually achieve sustainable growth. We may not be able to transplant it, but we can provide water, nutrients and maybe shade from a fierce sun. Therapy, it seems to me, exists to provide this healthy environment within which the wilting client can begin the process of receiving the nourishment (in the form of healthy relational experience) that can enable them, in time, to become a more fully functioning person.

Diagnosis

I have referred elsewhere (Bryant-Jefferies, 2003b) to the debate as to whether diagnosis can necessarily be trusted and empirical when it comes to mental health factors, drawing attention to Bozarth (2002) who refers to his own studies of particular diagnostic concepts which do not evidence the clustering of symptoms in a meaningful way (Bozarth, 1998) and to those of others in relation to schizophrenia (Bentall, 1990; Slade and Cooper, 1979), depression (Hallett, 1990; Weiner, 1989), agoraphobia (Hallam, 1983), borderline personality-disorder (Kutchins and Kirk, 1997) and panic disorder (Hallam, 1989).

The person-centred view of diagnosis generally regards it as a language associated with a medical model of working, and not always necessarily helpful or indeed descriptive beyond the person's behaviour. Yes, a particular set of symptoms may be usefully grouped under a heading – for instance, a certain level of being over-weight will be described as 'obesity' – but the risk is that the diagnosis assumes that the person has a set 'illness' that will be resolved by a specific 'treatment'. However, the reasons for an individual to develop problems associated with their eating pattern will be unique to them, will be the result of their own uniquely internalised meanings flowing from their own individual experiences.

It is important to acknowledge that symptomatology might be better seen as a kind of experiential flashing neon sign, drawing attention to the fact that something is wrong. If our treatment responses are simply concerned with turning off the flashing light because it is a problem to us, rather than seeking the underlying reason for which it is flashing, then we have a system that goes no further than symptom management. Whilst this may well have a part to play in bringing a client symptom relief, it should not be confused with actual treatment of the underlying cause.

Rogers questioned the value of psychological diagnosis. He argued that it could place the client's locus of value firmly outside themselves and definitely within the diagnosing 'expert', leaving the client at risk of developing tendencies of dependence and expectation that the 'expert' will have the responsibility of improving the client's situation (Rogers, 1951, p. 223). He also formulated the following propositional statements.

- Behaviour is caused, and the psychological cause of behaviour is a certain perception or a way of perceiving.
- The client is the only one who has the potentiality of knowing fully the dynamics of his perceptions and his behaviour.
- In order for behaviour to change, a change in perception must be *experienced*. Intellectual knowledge cannot substitute for this.
- The constructive forces which bring about altered perception, reorganisation of self, and relearning, reside primarily in the client, and probably cannot come from outside.
- Therapy is basically the experiencing of the inadequacies in old ways of perceiving, the experiencing of new and more accurate and adequate perceptions, and the recognition of significant relationship between perceptions.
- In a very meaningful and accurate sense, therapy *is* diagnosis, and this diagnosis is a process which goes on in the experience of the client, rather than in the intellect of the clinician (Rogers, 1951, pp. 221–3).

In a recent publication Steve Vincent has drawn together some valuable passages from Rogers in relation to the question of diagnosis, emphasising that '*therapist diagnosis, evaluation and prognosis clearly do not respect the inner resources of clients* and their potential and capacity for self-direction, as there is an obvious implication that actually the therapist, not the client, knows best' (Vincent, 2005). He then quotes a passage from Rogers from his earlier days, yet a statement that stands the test of time, sounding with great clarity an essential person-centred perspective on this issue.

If we can provide understanding of the way the client seems to himself at this moment, he can do the rest. The therapist must lay aside his pre-occupation with diagnosis and his diagnostic shrewdness, must discard his tendency to make professional evaluations, must cease his endeavours to formulate an accurate prognosis, must give up the temptation subtly to guide the individual, and must concentrate on one purpose only; that of providing deep understanding and acceptance of his attitudes consciously held at this moment by the client as he explores step by step into the dangerous areas which he has been denying to consciousness (Rogers, 1946).

Process of change from a person-centred perspective

Rogers was interested in understanding the process of change, what it was like, how it occurred and what experiences it brought to those involved – client and therapist. At different points he explored this. Embleton Tudor *et al.* (2004) point to a model consisting of 12 steps identified in 1942 (Rogers, 1942) and to his two later chapters on this topic (Rogers, 1951), and finally the seven-stage model (Rogers, 1967). He wrote of 'initially looking for elements which would mark or characterise change itself', however, what he experienced from his enquiry and research into the process of change he summarised as: 'individuals move, I began to see, not from fixity or homeostasis through change to a new fixity, though such a process is indeed possible. But much the more significant continuum is from fixity to changingness, from rigid structure to flow, from stasis to process. I formed the tentative hypothesis that perhaps the qualities of the client's expression at any one point might indicate his position on this continuum, where he stood in the process of change' (Rogers, 1967, p. 131).

Change, then, involves a movement from fixity to greater fluidity, from, we might say, a rigid set of attitudes and behaviours to a greater openness to experience, to variety and diversity. Change might be seen as having a certain liberating quality, a freeing up of the human being – his heart, mind, emotions – so that the person experiences themselves less of a fixed object and more of a conscious process. For the client who is seeking to resolve issues associated with a condition of obesity, part of this process will involve a loosening of the individual's identity that is strongly connected to their size and shape, or to the thoughts and feelings that they have about themselves that have driven them to gain excess weight. Until this is 'unfixed', if you like, it would seem reasonable to conclude that sustainable change might be extremely difficult to achieve.

The list that follows is taken from Rogers' summary of the process, indicating the changes that people will show (*see* Appendix 1).

1   This process involves a loosening of feelings.
2   This process involves a change in the manner of experiencing.
3   The process involves a shift from incongruence to congruence.
4   The process involves a change in the manner in which, and the extent to which the individual is able and willing to communicate himself in a receptive climate.
5   The process involves a loosening of the cognitive maps of experience.
6   There is a change in the individual's relationship to his problem.
7   There is a change in the individual's manner of relating (Rogers, 1967, pp. 156–8).

This is a very partial overview, the chapter in which he describes the process of change has much more detail and should be read in order to gain a clear grasp not only of the process as a whole, but of the distinctive features of each stage, as he saw it. Embleton Tudor *et al.* (2004) summarise this process in the following, and I think helpful, terms: 'a movement from fixity to fluidity, from closed to open, from tight to loose, and from afraid to accepting' (p. 47).

In Rogers' description of the process he makes the point that there were several types of process by which personality changes and that the process he described is one that is 'set in motion when the individual experiences himself as being fully received'. Does this process apply to all psychotherapies? Rogers indicated that more data were needed, adding that 'perhaps therapeutic approaches which place great stress on the cognitive and little on the emotional aspects of experience may set in motion an entirely different process of change'. In terms of whether this process of change would generally be viewed as desirable and that it would move the person in a valued direction, Rogers expressed the view that the valuing of a particular process of change was linked to social value judgements made by individuals and cultures. He pointed out that the process of change that he described could be avoided, simply by people 'reducing or avoiding those relationships in which the individual is fully received as he is'.

Rogers also took the view that change was unlikely to be rapid, making the point that many clients enter the therapeutic process at stage two, and leave at stage four, having during that period gained enough to feel satisfied. He suggested it would be 'very rarely, if ever, that a client who fully exemplified stage one would move to a point where he fully exemplified stage seven', and that if this did occur 'it would involve a matter of years' (Rogers, 1967, pp. 155–6). He wrote of how, at the outset, the threads of experience are discerned and understood separately by the client but as the process of change takes place, they move into 'the flowing peak moments of therapy in which all these threads become inseparably woven together.' He continues: 'in the new experiencing with immediacy which occurs at such moments, feeling and cognition interpenetrate, self is subjectively present in the experience, volition is simply the subjective following of a harmonious balance of organismic direction. Thus, as the process reaches this point the person becomes a unity of flow, of motion. He has changed, but what seems most significant, he has become an integrated process of changingness' (Rogers, 1967, p. 158).

It conjures up images of flowing movement, perhaps we should say purposeful flowing movement as being the essence of the human condition, a state that we each have the potential to become, or to realise. Is it something we generate or develop out of fixity, or does it exist within us all as a potential that we lose during our conditional experiencing in childhood? Are we discovering something new, or re-discovering something that was lost?

In the context of this book, we need to consider an holistic approach, with both eating/weight or size management behaviours and psychological processes interrelating (as they do) within the therapeutic process. Each will contribute to, and inform, the other process, a kind of feedback loop being generated, the system evolving and developing by feeding off the changes made and the experiences that those changes bring into awareness. The more satisfying to the person the experience of change is, the greater their motivation to pursue change further. In the context of the topic of this book, this process of psychological change, the re-balancing and integrating process then becomes evidenced through changes in eating behaviour.

Further person-centred perspectives

Person-centred theory affirms the importance of congruence, of being genuine, authentic, transparent. It seems to me that the relational component of the person-centred approach, based on the presence of the core conditions, is emerging strongly as a counter to the sense of isolation that frequently accompanies deep psychological and emotional problems. The concept of relational counselling was very much a driving force in the early development of the ideas that then developed into what we know as the person-centred approach. Of the counselling relationship Rogers wrote in 1942, 'The counselling relationship is one in which warmth of acceptance and absence of any coercion or personal pressure on the part of the counsellor permits the maximum expression of feelings, attitudes, and problems by the counselee . . . In the unique experience of complete emotional freedom within a well-defined framework the client is free to recognize and understand his impulses and patterns, positive and negative, as in no other relationship' (Rogers, 1942, pp. 113–4).

Working with a person or client who has an obese condition, like working with any other client about any other issue, is about forming therapeutic relationship and offering the client time and a space in which to explore, with increasing openness and authenticity, what they are experiencing. The person-centred counsellor will not take the perspective of being there to 'treat obesity', but to form a therapeutic relationship that will enable that client to experience constructive personality change that is self-directed through the process of the actualising tendency. As they become more authentically aware of themselves, and diminish the effects of 'conditions of worth' and re-evaluate their sense of self, they will very likely seek to change behaviours so as to establish new ones that more closely satisfy the needs of their changing sense of self. As the causes of their overeating are recognised and understood, and begin to loosen their grip, the eating behaviour will change, and with a likelihood that it will be in a sustainable way because it is driven by psychological and emotional change which, itself, is the result of the actualising tendency operating within a person-centred therapeutic experience.

I am extremely encouraged by the increasing interest in the PCA, the growing amount of material being published, and the realisation that relationship is a key factor in positive therapeutic outcome. There is currently much debate about theoretical developments within the person-centred world and its application. Discussions on the theme of Rogers' therapeutic conditions presented by various key members of the person-centred community have recently been published (Bozarth and Wilkins, 2001; Haugh and Merry 2001; Wyatt, 2001; Wyatt and Sanders, 2002). Mearns and Thorne have produced a timely publication revising and developing key aspects of person-centred theory (2000). Wilkins has produced a book that addresses most effectively many of the criticisms levelled against person-centred working (2003) and Embleton Tudor *et al.* (2004) an introduction to the person-centred approach that places the theory and practice within a contemporary context. Recently, Howard Kirschenbaum (Carl Rogers' biographer) published an article entitled 'The current status of Carl Rogers and the person-centred approach'. In his research for this article he noted that from 1946–86 there were 84 books, 64 chapters and 456 journal articles published on Carl Rogers and the person-centred approach. In contrast, from 1987–2004 there were 141 books, 174 book chapters and 462 journal articles published. A clear trend towards more publications and, presumably, more readership and interest in the approach. Also, he noted that there were now some 50 person-centred publications available around the world, mostly journals and there are now person-centred organisations in 18 countries, and 20 organisations overall. He also draws attention to the large body of research demonstrating the effectiveness of person-centred therapy, concluding that the person-centred approach is 'alive and well' and appears to be experiencing 'something of a revival, both in professional activity and academic respectability' (Kirschenbaum, 2005). There are many other books, and perhaps there is a need now for a comprehensive database of all person- or client-centred books to be made available to all training organisations and person-centred networks. And perhaps it already exists.

This is obviously a very brief introduction to the theory of the approach. Person-centred theory continues to develop as practitioners and theoreticians consider its application in various fields of therapeutic work and extend our theoretical understanding of developmental and therapeutic processes. At times it feels like it has become more than just individuals, rather it feels like a group of colleagues, based around the world, working together to penetrate deeper towards a more complete theory of the human condition, and this includes people from the many traditions and schools of thought. Person-centred or client-centred theory and practice has a key role in this process. Theories are being revisited and developed, new ideas speculated upon, new media explored for presenting the core values and philosophy of the person-centred approach. It is an exciting time.

PART I

Steve confronts being overweight

Steve nodded, 'I suppose my size has been a major factor in shaping me, the person, me, Steve, you know?' He went quiet, the words 'fat bastard' came to mind, he'd been called that a few times. On a good day, he laughed, brushed it off, he could even make a joke of it himself, though if he was really honest with himself he would have to admit that at some level it hurt. On a bad day? Two reactions. Want to get away, hideaway, though that happened less rarely. More often on a bad day he'd want to punch the lights out of whoever had said it.

CHAPTER 1

Counselling session 1: forming a therapeutic relationship

Steve sat and looked at the posters on the walls in the waiting room. The chairs were small and it made him quite conscious of his size. Anywhere that he went he overflowed the seat and could sense the irritation of others. His attitude had always been 'fuck them', but behind that there was a discomfort that he rarely let anyone else see.

He had been large for as long as he could remember and it felt as though it had been OK and acceptable until recently, until all the fuss about obesity and people who were larger were suddenly a cause of excess costs to the health service. His GP had been mentioning his weight for years, but he had chosen to ignore it. Sometimes it might make him think, cause him to hesitate when he was contemplating what to eat, but generally he brushed it aside. His attitude was very much that of it being no one else's business what he ate.

Now, however, his blood pressure was definitely up and the doctor was expressing serious concerns. He had also had experiences of breathlessness which had left him feeling quite dizzy and disorientated on occasions. He was being monitored closely and the choice was very much a case of lose weight or we will have to put you on medication. He didn't like tablets. He liked to feel he was in control. But he knew that the tablets probably wouldn't help the breathlessness anyway, and that was what had concerned him most. It was something tangible, it had stopped him and made him think – 35 years old and breathless. He couldn't carry on like that, and yet he didn't like feeling picked on because of his size. He reacted against that.

As he sat waiting for his appointment with the counsellor, his eyes focused on a poster – highlighting the damage to health caused by obesity. Didn't see those on the walls a few years back. But the way it was written, it seemed so critical, blaming people for putting on weight. OK, so he had decided to build himself up, but he had always had a healthy appetite – that was what his mum had always said – and, well, he just spent a lot of time eating. He liked eating.

It can get forgotten that for many people who have a weight problem, eating is something that they enjoy. Generally people don't like to give up or cut back on what brings them pleasure. People make choices because it gives them a benefit. We make choices and develop behaviours to satisfy needs. Eating is, for many people, a way of satisfying a range of needs: to offset boredom, to make themselves feel big, for the sensation of feeling full, to make themselves feel they are less attractive, and there are many more. And what you eat, or where you eat, can be an indicator of affluence and signify a form of status, or to be seen to be in touch with the latest fashion, to be where your friends are.

John was sitting in the counselling room. He had been a counsellor for a number of years, and had recently become interested in working with people who had weight problems. He now worked two sessions a week at the local hospital. It was a new area that was under development and he was excited by it, although he was aware that many of the issues underlying a person's eating pattern and weight gain were those that he encountered generally as a counsellor: sexual abuse and bullying being two areas that arose frequently, together with symptoms of depression.

He noted the time and went out to look for his new client – Steve. He was always mindful of his approach. The difficulty was that in general he would know who his client was before they knew him – their size would make them stand out.Yet he also wanted to normalise things, and if there were a number of people in the waiting area, he would call out his client's name without fixing his eyes specifically on the person who it seemed highly likely was going to be his client. It wasn't that it was a right or wrong way to approach it, just the way that he had developed.

He went into the waiting room, and called out his client's name. Steve had looked up when John had entered. He heard his name mentioned and met his eyes. 'That's me.'

'Hi, would you like to come through?' He was always careful not to announce himself as 'the counsellor'; the client might have met someone that they knew, but didn't want them to know why they were attending.

Steve followed John along the corridor to the counselling room. The first thing he noticed were that the chairs were large and accommodating. 'Where shall I sit?'

This attention to detail communicates something to clients. Of course, how the client will receive it will be up to them, but for the person-centred counsellor what is important is that such details are an expression of their wish to communicate respect and warm acceptance to their clients as persons with their particular set of needs.

'Whichever. Up to you.'

Steve sat in the chair opposite to where he was standing as he had come through the door.

'So, you've been referred to me by your doctor. I need to say something before we start about confidentiality, although I know we sent you a leaflet describing what this means, as well as what counselling offers.'

'Sure.'

John informed Steve as to the nature of confidentiality and its limits, and checked that Steve felt informed about what he was being offered.

Steve said that he was.

Explaining the scope of confidentiality and providing information so that the client can give informed consent to receive counselling is important. It can feel rather administrative in that it is an outside agenda being imposed on the client, however, where a client is referred for something, rather than it being their own informed choice, they do need to know what they are being offered, and for what purpose.

'Great, I have to mention all this, and I have to be sure that you are giving consent to treatment.' John had the momentary thought to himself of the fact that he didn't think of counselling as a treatment, but that within the health service that was the language that was used. As a person-centred counsellor he saw himself offering contact and relationship which he believed encouraged clients to become more accurately and authentically self-aware. For him, working with people on eating issues so often related back to experiences in their lives. People developed particular eating patterns for reasons, they had their own specific meaning that they attached to it, and to themselves as a person who had extra weight. If people could resolve the psychological factors he believed very strongly that the eating pattern could then change, and most importantly, change in a sustainable way.

'Sure, that's fine.' Steve made himself comfortable, although he was aware of feeling a bit anxious and uncertain, not being sure quite what would happen next.

'So, where would you like to begin? What's going on for you?'

Steve took a deep breath. 'Well, I don't know how much of a problem I've got, but the doctor thinks that I have.' Steve didn't want to openly admit to the problem, or that his eating was causing a problem, he didn't want someone judging him as having made himself 'unwell', which was how he felt lots of people viewed people with obesity issues.

'Mhmm, the doctor thinks you have a problem, but you're not so sure.'

'I mean, I've always been big, long as I can remember and, well, I don't like anyone telling me there's something wrong with me – makes me feel like, I don't know, I'm suddenly a problem.'

'So you don't like anyone telling you something's wrong, you don't like being made to feel that you're suddenly a problem, yes?'

Steve nodded. 'That's right. I don't like it and I won't put up with it.'

'People telling you that you're a problem, well, you're not going to stand for it.'

'No, no I'm not.' Although Steve felt quite tense as he spoke and had strong feelings about this; he was also relaxing a little into the session and into a dialogue with John. 'I mean, OK, so, yeah, so I'm big, but I've always been big, so what? So I have some health issues. OK. But I don't want people to start blaming me.'

This series of empathic responses has meant that the client has moved more fully into his feelings and that they are becoming more present in his physical state and through his tone of words. Empathic understanding is not conveyed by the person-centred therapist to achieve this, they offer empathic responses in order to convey their understanding of what the client is telling them. The effect will be as it is. Often, however, it will enable clients to engage more fully with their feelings or thoughts because they have felt heard and respected, and either feel they can disclose more, or simply connect with feelings that demand to be expressed.

'Yes, I think I understand, it's more the sense of people blaming you, and I suppose – and this is a word that is present for me – a sense of people "judging you".' John used the word 'judging' not because it was a common feeling among clients in these kinds of situations, but because it arose within him strongly in response to what Steve was saying, and the way he was saying it.

'I don't like being judged. I'm not fat, I'm large.'

'And large is what you have been for as long as you can remember. You don't feel fat and you don't want to be judged. That all sounds pretty clear to me.'

Steve nodded, thinking to himself that at least he'd made that clear. He wanted to get things straight. Make sure this guy John knew who he was talking to and what he was saying.

It is worth considering whether the tone and content of what the client is saying is in some way linked to the fact that his counsellor is male. Might he talk differently if the counsellor was a woman? Would this have been more, or less, therapeutically valuable? All we can say is that it would have been different and, from a person-centred perspective, what is important is that a therapeutic relationship is established. Nevertheless, certain gender mixes will have particular meanings for clients.

Another issue is the size and shape of the counsellor. Would it help if they, too, were large? Or does it make little difference? Does a difference in size encourage or discourage a client to express him or herself in different ways? It will vary from person to person. It may prove helpful for the counsellor to acknowledge any awareness that they have of difference, but only if it emerges in the context of what the client is experiencing and describing, otherwise it would simply direct the client towards the counsellor's awareness.

Steve lapsed into silence and John stayed with it, respecting it. His sense was that perhaps Steve had said what he needed to for the moment and that he had felt heard, and therefore now knew he didn't need to say it again, but maybe wasn't sure what to say next. This was, in fact, quite true. Steve did feel heard, and it was actually a rather new experience to him, at least, it was from someone who wasn't large like he was. Some of his friends were large and they understood what he felt, and they generally felt the same, but anyone who wasn't his size, he'd usually sense that they weren't really listening or understanding. Over the years he'd become quite sensitive to peoples' reactions, you could see it in their eyes. And they had 'judgement' written all over them. Pissed him off.

Steve's thoughts were back with his doctor, who he also felt was quite judgemental. Seemed to be telling him what to do, how to live his life. Well, he'd done what he'd said, he'd come to see this counsellor, and now he was wondering what next. He'd told him how he felt and, yeah, he felt the guy had understood. Well, that was something. Now what?

John felt that he would acknowledge the silence and give Steve an opportunity to say what was happening for him. He was always reluctant to break in on a silence, and yet he also knew that in silences early on in a counselling relationship, and in this context where it seemed that a client had said their piece and then ground to a halt, he felt it was helpful to acknowledge what was happening. 'I hope that I've heard what you had to say just then, Steve, and maybe you're wondering what next?'

'I guess it happens a lot?' Steve thought that John was making some standard response.

'It can do. It can take a while sometimes, and silences happen, and it gives people a chance to think about what they're experiencing.'

'I guess I want someone to give me some ideas, you know, but not tell me what to do. I like to make my own mind up about things.'

'Sure, feel you're in control, you decide what you want to do.'

'Yeah, that's important. I guess it's the same for most people.'

'People can be similar, but they're all uniquely different as well.'

'I guess you see all kinds of people, you must see people in a really bad way?'

John acknowledged to himself the switch of focus and content. Steve was now asking him questions.

As a person-centred counsellor, John will want to feel that he can honour his client's question. Whilst in some approaches a response might be to ask why the question is important, the person-centred counsellor is more likely to want to respond openly and transparently. After all, he is seeking,

> through congruence, to establish greater congruence within the therapeu-
> tic relationship and the client.

'All kinds of people, all kinds of needs.'

Steve felt he wanted to pursue his questioning. He wanted to know a little more about this guy. OK, he'd read the leaflet, but he wasn't very big himself. Did he really know much about obesity? Did he really? And then he questioned why he was thinking these things. What did it matter anyway, he was here, he'd done what the doctor had requested. It was up to this counsellor to sort him out. 'But you see people about eating – lots of people?'

'Yes, I do.'

'And they are helped?'

John nodded. 'Yes, I believe so.'

'You mean they lose weight?'

'Sometimes, and sometimes they focus more on other areas of themselves or their lives, but usually to things that are connected.'

'But not everyone loses weight?'

'Not everyone wants to.'

'So you only help people who want to lose weight?'

'No, no I don't. Sometimes it's about helping people to get to know themselves better so that they might begin to want to lose weight themselves.'

'Well, I've got to lose a bit.' Steve was slightly surprised to hear himself say that. It had sort of been said unintentionally, like a normal kind of conversation.

John noted the ownership by Steve of his having to lose some weight himself. He wasn't going to over-empathise which might have the effect of Steve backing off, he'd maintain his sensitivity to Steve feeling able to acknowledge his own need.

> Can a counsellor over-empathise? It may seem a strange concept, but when a client tentatively says something, or says something that is indicative of a shift of perception, the counsellor needs to respond carefully and sensitively. The client has made something visible in the relationship that may be quite fragile, or at least, it may be a perception or an experience that is either new to the client, or new in the sense of it not having been shared before with another person.

'Mhmm, you kind of feel you've got to lose a bit yourself.' By not using the word 'weight', which Steve has also not used, it lightens the response. The word 'weight' could be emotive. There's no need to say it. Had he done so it could have been an instance of over-empathising and Steve might have retreated away from his acknowledgement.

'Doctor thinks so.'

'Doctor does, but you're not so sure.'

'No, I know he's right. I mean, you know, look at me. I'm big, I know it, but I don't really want to admit it.'

'Sure, it's not easy to accept, especially in the context of it being what a doctor is telling you.'

Steve smiled. That was true enough. 'He's been telling me for years, but, well, I guess now I'm feeling different because of it.'

'Different because of ...?' John was unsure to what Steve was referring and wanted to clarify his understanding.

'Different because I get the episodes when I get breathless. I mean, I suppose I've had something similar for a while, but, well, I've sort of ignored it, like you do. But, well, he's telling me that it's serious, that it's because of the strain on my heart. And, well, he says my blood pressure's too high. It's been high for a while, but, well, now he says I have to do something about it.'

John was struck by the tone of Steve's voice. It sounded somehow more accepting, his tone had changed from the start of the session. He felt that perhaps there was now the beginning of the relationship he knew needed to form between them.

Although the content of the dialogue has been important; in fact all that is communicated is the preliminary stage in a relationship-building process. Two men – one a 'client', one a 'counsellor' are sitting together in a room, establishing some degree of rapport. It may be established quickly – sometimes client and counsellor 'click', sometimes it takes a while.

It is important that the relationship is given time to develop. This is particularly relevant in person-centred counselling because it is, in essence, relationship counselling. It is the establishing and the experiencing of the therapeutic relationship, governed by the presence of the 'necessary and sufficient conditions for constructive personality change', that are the crucial factors. The information exchanged is interesting and useful, but at this stage in the counselling process it is a kind of vehicle through which relationship is established.

'So, your doctor is quite clear, in his view you have to do something about it.'

Steve nodded. And part of him knew the doctor was right, but he didn't want to be told what to do, didn't want to feel pushed into something. He had friends who were large and they didn't seem to be being told to change. Why was he being singled out?

'So he says. But it doesn't seem fair. I know people, older than me, bigger then me, they're not being told to change what they eat, or to go and do some exercise. Why me?'

'So you feel, what, picked on, that it doesn't seem fair, why you when others seem to eat more and are larger, and they don't get told to change?'

Picked on. Those words took Steve back to his past. Bastards, he thought to himself. He pushed the memories aside. 'That's right. Only me. Why me?'

John noted that Steve had twice asked 'why me?'. His sense was that clearly Steve did not have, but desperately wanted, an answer. And, of course, there wasn't one, other than the fact that for whatever reason his health was being affected now. Maybe his friends had also been told to do something but were keeping it to themselves. But to introduce that would be to take Steve away from the question that is pulling at him: 'why me?'.

'Why you? Why do you seem to be the one affected like this?' John nodded as he spoke, and sat tight-lipped after he had spoken, allowing the question to remain present in the room, and in the relationship. It felt like it sat there, yes, in Steve's head and to some degree in his own, but it also felt it was sitting between them in the room. He decided to voice his experience as it felt quite strong, and clearly was linked to their therapeutic dialogue.

When does a person-centred counsellor voice some internal experience that they are having when they are with a client? We need to be clear, first of all, that the meaning of congruence is not 'I feel/think therefore I tell my client'.

Counsellors experience all kinds of things in therapy sessions, some of which are connected to the therapeutic process, some of which are their own stuff bubbling through. The counsellor has to decide what is appropriate to disclose. Is it likely to be therapeutically helpful? Is it pressing and urgent, yet clearly not connected to something specific within the counsellor's own experience? The counsellor may not always get it right. There is something about the tone of what has become present within the counsellor's awareness. Whenever this occurs, it is best to offer the experience tentatively.

There needs to be a sense of connection with the client, as if the client and counsellor's frames of reference have overlapped or merged to some degree, however minimal. Bringing in an experience that has arisen within the counsellor's awareness, if not done tentatively, could cut right across the therapeutic process and cause great disturbance, confusion and disorientation within the client.

'I'm kind of sitting here with a feeling of this "why me?" present here between us, waiting for us to work it out, or come up with some answer.'

For Steve it felt much more present in his own head, but there was something about what John had said that he appreciated. As though the question was perhaps not his alone to answer. Truth was, he didn't have an answer and it felt like he wasn't quite so alone with it while John had been speaking. Maybe he could try and think of it that way as well. 'I don't know why, and I sort of do want to know, and I don't. Knowing why might be bad news.'

'You don't want bad news.'

'Feels like I already have that, don't think I want any more.'

'The knowing you are experiencing health problems, that's bad news enough, you mean?'

Steve nodded. He sat quietly, mulling over what had just been said. Did he really want to know why? Did he need to? Truth was, the more he thought about it, he didn't, it seemed to be how it was, much as he didn't like it and didn't want to accept it, much as he wanted his high blood pressure and breathlessness to be caused by something else. 'I guess I can't avoid it. It's how it is and I have to deal with it.'

'Can't avoid the facts, you mean, and you have no choice but to deal with the implications.' John noted a certain tone of ambivalence, clearly Steve was unsure what he wanted, and that wasn't unusual, particularly at first when a person was faced with the view that their weight was a problem and needed addressing. Some people felt relief, it sort of made it easier to talk about, but other people were more ambivalent and guarded. A lot depended on the client's own perspective. Some would be more ready to contemplate the need for change than others, and some would be more uncomfortable with the whole idea.

Yes, Steve thought to himself, as he took a deep breath and let the air out slowly. He was looking down at his stomach and thinking, 'it's no good, you're going to have to go'. He couldn't imagine himself being anything other than how he was. It seemed like he was being asked to lose part of himself, yes, become less of who he was. He was used to being himself. That seemed a daft thought. He was himself, of course he was used to being who he was and how he was. Now he had to somehow be different, do things differently. He shook his head, still in thought and still in silence.

Clients will have mixed feelings and will find it hard to imagine how they would be with less weight. They may have only experienced themselves as being large for many years, perhaps for most of their life. It will be a part of their identity and it will not be easy for them to change this, or, indeed, to feel that they want to change this. The thought of being thinner is in a sense unthinkable, it is not who or what they are.

The counsellor must be able to hear this if this is what the client experiences and communicates, possibly through apparent ambivalence to change. For many people it will feel easier to contemplate staying as they are, rather than facing the uncertainty of change. It is a difficult decision. It is a sensitive area and the counsellor must be empathic to their client as they explore what they think and feel about change, and the implications that it will have, and the thoughts and feelings that it will bring up.

John watched Steve looking down and shaking his head. He guessed that he was deep in thought and he felt he would not disturb whatever process was underway. He knew there were times when it was right to respond to a silence by acknowledging it in some way; whereas at other times the therapeutic response was to show empathy for the silence by communicating silence back. Of course, it wasn't really a silence. It was simply a period of time in which the client was choosing not to verbally communicate anything to the counsellor, but the reality was far from a silence. There was probably too much going on within Steve's thoughts and feeling for it to be a silence in the sense of being empty and devoid of movement.

Steve sat wondering just how it would be. How would he begin to make any changes? What would his wife think? She'd probably be pleased, she had said a few times that his weight had gone up quite a lot recently. And he also had moments in which he wasn't aware of thinking anything, blank moments as though his mind had given up for a few seconds. He knew the doctor was right, however much he tried to find arguments against what he had said. His weight had been steadily going up these last two years or so. And yet he still didn't really want to accept it. Just wanted to live his life, do what he did the way he did, he'd always been happy like that.

Steve had lost track of time as he sat thinking about it all. John, meanwhile, sat quietly, maintaining his attention and focus on Steve. He wanted to be sure of being present for him should he wish to express anything verbally or non-verbally. Looking at him now, he had a frown on his face, and he looked so intent, so serious. And of course, he was having to contemplate a very serious issue. It seemed that his health was at risk, there was now actual evidence that Steve had and was experiencing. Sometimes that made a big difference. Telling someone that if they carried on the way they were then, one day, such and such would happen, never really had the same impact as someone being told that what they were now experiencing was linked to a particular behaviour.

John was aware of what he was feeling for Steve. Yes, there was a quality of sympathy present, a feeling of, poor guy, having to face up to the need to make what for him must be a significant change. Was it right to feel sympathy? He often heard people saying you're supposed to show empathy. But he didn't agree. He wasn't going to start saying 'poor thing', but he couldn't hide sympathy that would be in his eyes when clients disclosed difficult and challenging experiences, or the need to face up to something that was awful and they knew they were going to struggle with. For John, sympathy was a quality of the heart and what human beings needed, in their moments of despair, as a sense of heartfelt responses from others.

A person-centred counsellor will wish to be authentically present with their clients, and if a profound sense of sympathy emerges within them in response to their empathic connection and therapeutic relationship with their client, then they will not try and hide it from them. They will allow it to be present, acknowledging it for themselves and making the choice as to whether it will be appropriate and helpful to own it and voice it to the client along the lines of, 'hearing you say that leaves me feeling ...', and if the wonder is there, the counsellor might voice, 'and I wonder if that feeling has meaning for you?', or something similar.

If you are unsure about sympathy, ask yourself if, when you disclose to someone an experience that is painful to you, you feel acknowledged by your own sense of the other person's sympathy – the look in their eyes, their facial expression, and what they say and how they say it. Sympathy is a natural human response, and in moments of despair we are strengthened by the presence of heartfelt, human responses around us and towards us. This is true in therapy as it is in life. (And therapy is, of course, part of life though some may think it so precious as to be separate or different.)

Steve took another deep breath. 'I know I have to change, and I don't want to accept it.' He looked up, and met John's eye contact. He noticed the look on John's face. He looked like he understood. He looked as though he was with him in some way. He didn't look as distant as he had seemed earlier in the session. He looked as though he cared. He wasn't sure what to make of it, but didn't try. He wasn't feeling like thinking.

It was John's turn to take a deep breath. 'Yeah, you know you have to, but ...' He didn't finish the sentence, he didn't have to. He sensed that Steve knew he was conveying an appreciation of what he, Steve, was feeling.

Steve took another deep breath. 'Bugger.' He looked at the clock. 'Nearly time to go.'

John nodded.

Steve shook his head. He felt his focus move. 'None of this is what I expected.'

'No?'

'I mean, I wasn't sure what to expect, but nothing like this. I thought you'd be asking me lots of questions.'

John smiled. 'Not how I work.'

'I can see that. But you haven't even asked me what my weight is.'

John shrugged, 'no, I guess I haven't.'

'And yet I feel, I don't know, I'm not sure what I'm feeling or thinking at the moment.'

'Counselling can feel quite disorientating, particularly to begin with. You spend time with feelings and thoughts and they can have a profound effect.'

'Well, I don't know what to do next, but something's been going on.'

'Just look after yourself once you have left, take a bit of time if you can to collect your thoughts and then get yourself gradually back into the day.'

Steve nodded again.

'So, I want to check whether this feels helpful, and whether you want to come back, and if yes, decide how soon.'

'Well, because I'm self-employed I can fit myself around it, though first thing or last is best as it means it won't disrupt my work as much.'

'Sure.' John checked the diary. 'Early is probably best for me, 9.15 am is my first appointment slot. How soon do you want to come back?'

'What's normal?'

'Depends. Some people come weekly, some fortnightly, others longer.'

'I feel I need to think about it all a bit more. How about in two weeks?'

'That's fine, time to think about it and we'll take it from there.'

'And there's nothing you're going to tell me to do?'

'What do you want to do, Steve?'

Steve tightened his lips. 'I need to shed a few pounds.'

John nodded, 'mhmm, you need to shed a few pounds.' He felt that this was important, not simply from what Steve was saying, but the way he was saying it. There was a kind of calm – or was it more resigned? – acceptance. But he trusted Steve with that knowledge, and that he would do with it whatever he felt he needed, and was able, to. No point in pushing him. Yes, he would encourage him, but encourage him to be real, be honest with himself. His subjective sense was that changes rooted in people being honest with themselves were far more likely to succeed than changes imposed on them by others.

The session ended and Steve left, feeling strangely more accepting of his need to lose weight. It wasn't that he hadn't known before, he sort of had, but he didn't like being told what to do. He reacted against it. John wasn't telling him. But he knew he had to do something. He didn't like it. He felt that John had listened to him. He wasn't sure exactly what John knew about weight, whether he'd been overweight himself. He hadn't thought about that much in the session. Maybe it didn't matter. He didn't know.

Meanwhile, John sat back in his chair and pondered on the session. He was conscious of his size, he was a lot smaller than Steve. It was something that he was aware of with clients sometimes, and on some occasions more so than on others. He suspected he was more aware of it with male clients coming to discuss issues around obesity. There seemed more scope for comparison. He wondered if it was the same with women with obesity who saw female counsellors. He could imagine that could be the case, for some people, but not all. And whatever attitude people had it would be the result of their own individual and unique experiences and the meanings they attributed to size and shape. He began to write his notes.

Points for discussion

- How do you ensure that your clients understand the limits of confidentiality and that they are informed as to what they are giving consent?
- Evaluate John's application of the person-centred approach in this first session.
- What were the key moments in the session?
- How would you relate the content of this session to the 'processes of change' described in Appendices 1 and 2?
- Would you have responded differently had you been Steve's counsellor and, if so, how and why? Justify these differences theoretically.

- What role do you feel the presence of sympathetic reactions in the counsellor have on the effectiveness of the therapeutic process?
- If you were the counsellor what would you take to supervision from this session?
- Write notes for this session.

CHAPTER 2

Counselling session 2: anger, acceptance and planning change

It had not been a good fortnight for Steve. Somehow that first counselling session seemed to have made things worse. He seemed to feel he was eating more. He wasn't sure why, but just found he spent the week thinking more about food and not being able to distract himself. Yes, he knew he had to do something, he was uncomfortable with it, with everything. At times, yes, that was it, he just felt uncomfortable with himself, with life, the universe, everything. As a result things had not been easy at home. His wife told him he was 'going round like a bear with a sore head, and a fat bear at that'.

As mentioned before, people don't like changing something that they enjoy. It is uncomfortable, unsettling. At the outset, people can start eating more, eating on the discomfort that has become more present for them as they feel the need to accept they have to make changes.

Others will eat more because their sense of change being inevitable means they feel they need a 'final fling' as it were; eat all the things they know they may have to give up or cut back on, a kind of goodbye 'taster', as it were.

He'd reacted. He knew he shouldn't have done, but he did, and he pushed her. Of course, with his weight what seemed a small push wasn't and she had fallen over the end of the sofa. An argument had ensued. Now, well, now the tension had passed although he was aware that she seemed more wary of him, more distant. It hadn't helped their relationship. He felt angry with himself, angry with John, and generally pissed off. He had thought of not coming, but felt he wanted to say something. And there was something pulling him back that he hadn't really got clarity on, and it was linked to the fact that John had listened, had seemed to understand. But that had been pushed aside by his concern for how he had reacted in the two weeks, and his sense that the counselling was to blame.

'Well, I've eaten more these two weeks so I'm not sure that this counselling has helped at all, in fact, I think it's made it worse.'

'Mhmm, so what you experienced here two weeks ago you feel has made you eat more?'

'Yeah, left me just, I don't know, but I thought it might help me.'

'So you felt it was unhelpful.'

'Yes. Well, not at the time, no, but since, yes, hasn't done me any good at all.'

'OK, so at the time that last session seemed helpful, but the past two weeks have been worse and you feel that the counselling session had something to do with it, that's how it feels?'

The counsellor stays close to what the client is saying, and avoiding any defensiveness as a result of the client conveying criticism of their first session. The client is allowed to say what he feels, and it is received and heard. Connection is being made on a topic and towards feelings that are very much present for the client.

It is important for a client to feel able to express critical thoughts and feelings. A defensive reaction might leave the client thinking twice about doing that another time, and their potential for congruent expression is therefore blocked.

'Yes, it is, and I've been irritable and angry, and pissed off with my wife, Jackie, as well.'

John nodded, gradually making his responses slightly more intense in tone, matching the tone of what Steve was saying, empathising with the way he was speaking as much as with what he was saying.

'So, it's all left you angry, irritable, and pissed off with your wife.'

'I mean, if I want to eat what I want, why the fuck shouldn't I?'

'You want to eat, it's your decision, like you said before, you don't want anyone telling you what to do.'

'No, I fucking don't.'

'You want to make your own fucking choices, yeah, not choices someone else tells you that you make?' The tone was intensifying even more.

'I do, I fucking well do.' Steve thumped the arm of the chair; it was quite a blow.

'Yeah.' John nodded. 'Yeah.' John and Steve were now looking at each other; Steve having looked intently at John the moment he had hit the arm of the chair. There was anger, but there was something else John could see in Steve's eyes, and it looked to him like in the midst of all the anger and frustration was a man knowing he needed help, but who sure wasn't going to ask for it. Although by coming to the counselling, in a sense he was doing just that.

'You look angry Steve . . . , and more than angry.' He maintained his eye contact and focus. Not feeling intimidated, even though he acknowledged Steve was a big man and he was sure that if he really lost it he could do a lot of damage. But he wasn't going to get anxious about that. Steve felt angry and needed to show that anger. John wasn't going to try and get in the way of it. Yes, he was going to hopefully let Steve know that his anger was accepted and acceptable.

The counsellor warmly accepts Steve's feelings and his need to express them. There may come a point at which safety issues need to be raised, but not unless this is a congruent expression of genuine concern. And the counsellor will wish to be clear as to what that concern is, and why. Otherwise, the client may well perceive that their anger is unacceptable.

What the person-centred counsellor wants to convey is that the feelings of anger are perfectly acceptable, it is a matter of how they are expressed and what might be the limit to acceptability should the client damage furniture, the counsellor or themselves. Therapists need to be clear as to what is acceptable, and to be able to convey this to clients, and why, should the need arise.

Would the client have engaged with and expressed his anger in the same way had he been with a female counsellor? And, if so, how might she respond and to what effect? Again, differences of gender might impact on the process. This is not a good or bad, better or worse issue. It is simply a fact of life. However, the intention will be to communicate unconditional positive regard and empathic understanding, to maintain a state of congruence and of integration in the therapeutic relationship, in the hope that these are perceived by the client.

Steve heard the first part of John's response and he was saying, too bloody right, to himself as he then heard John finish the sentence. More than angry. More than angry. Yes, he wasn't just angry, bloody angry; there were other feelings as well, under the anger. He could feel them now. One of them was fear. He didn't like it. He didn't want to experience it. He certainly didn't want to show it to another man.

Again, the client is allowed to go with his feelings and express them. The counsellor maintains contact through his empathy, and uses tone of voice and language to convey his sense of the strength of feeling present. Again, it is important for the client to feel he or she can voice their feelings. As a result they become more present and, in this case, the client identifies a feeling that he doesn't want to make visible to his counsellor, not at this stage in the relationship. And that is fine.

The person-centred counsellor is not going to try and pull feelings out of the client, that is not their job, and it would not be congruent to person-centred theory and practice. The counsellor offers the therapeutic conditions, staying open and warm towards the client, allowing the client's own process to take them where they need to go, and to express what they need and feel able to say.

They both sat in silence. 'I guess I've got to find my own way to do things.'
'What do you want, Steve?'
Steve snorted and blinked. 'Have a long and healthy life.'
'Yeah. That's important, huh?'
Steve nodded. 'Yeah.' He swallowed. 'Yeah, that's what I want, and ...'
  He paused, tightening his lips for a few moments. John did not interrupt but
  waited for Steve to continue. '... and that's where I'm stuck, I guess.'
'Feel stuck, stuck trying to achieve that long and healthy life.'
Steve nodded. 'I know I've got to lose weight, but I don't like being told.'
'Yeah, you want to make that decision yourself, in your own way, in your own
  time.'
'Not sure about time, I think maybe time's running out. I mean, I've had more
  episodes of breathlessness these past two weeks. I've got to do something.'
  He paused and looked up. 'You can get your jaws clamped, can't you?'
'Probably; is that how bad it seems?'
'I think so. But I don't want that, unless I really have to. I've got to learn to eat
  less, haven't I?'
'Yeah, get a sense of what you are eating and drinking now, and then think about
  what you can cut back on.'
'Yeah', Steve sighed, 'yeah, I have to.'
'So you really feel that you need to make a change, it's a case of how and what?'

The tone has changed. Perhaps the client felt heard enough in his anger and
frustration to now risk sharing his fear. He hasn't called it that but by being
asked what he wanted – which wasn't a directly empathic response though
perhaps it picked up on the reflective shift – the client has spoken of wanting
'a long and healthy life'. And from this generalisation he is now moving
towards acknowledging specifics that need to change to help ensure that
he achieves this. He is worried; the symptoms are distressing him, but he
doesn't want to show or share that distress with another man. The counsellor seeks to maintain empathy and an attitude of warm acceptance, seeking
to find that 'alongside' place beside his client.

'Yeah, and I guess it means the fatty foods, the chips, all the things that I probably
  don't need, but, well, like, you know?'
'I know. You eat a lot of chips and fatty foods.'
'Fried breakfast every day, fish and chips a couple of times a week, and, yeah,
  quite a stack of sandwiches at lunch-time as well.'
'So, need to try and reduce that down a bit. Any thoughts on what you can see
  yourself not eating, or eating less of?'
Steve thought about it. 'I suppose, I don't know, I'm so used to a large breakfast.
  I couldn't cut that out.'
'OK, could you cut it down?'

Steve thought about his breakfasts; bacon, eggs, sausages, fried bread, and toast. Lots of butter. Tea with lots of sugar. Didn't look good, he knew that. He told John what he had.

'Can you cut anything out? Has it all got to be fried?'

'I suppose the fried bread's not good, is it, and the butter? But it's the quantity as well.'

'Two eggs?'

'Sometimes three.'

'Can you reduce that a bit?'

Steve nodded. 'I guess I can try.'

'I mean, it's about taking it slowly. You know you need to cut back and my sense is that you want to as well. You've got a reason to, you want a long and healthy life, yeah?'

Steve nodded.

The counsellor has shifted into more of a motivational mode, focusing on the detail of what the client is saying and looking for what might be changed. From a person-centred perspective he has, in a sense, got ahead of the client, although the client is talking in the context of wanting to change in order to give himself that chance of a long and healthy life.

Empathy is not only about responses to what has been said, there is a contextual quality as well. It can be argued that the counsellor is responding to the context of the client wanting to change, so he focuses on that in his responses to his client.

'So something has to give. But make sure what you change is the thing you genuinely feel you can do.'

'I know. I need to cut back. It's going to look a small plateful.'

John nodded. He could see the uncomfortable look on Steve's face. 'A small plateful, not a comfortable prospect?'

Steve shook his head again. 'No, but I have to start somewhere, and maybe that's as good a place as any. I need to talk to Jackie. I know she'd be happy to cook less – she moans about the cost as well.'

'I guess it will need you to work together on it.'

Steve nodded. 'I know. We're not getting on too well at the moment, but I think she'll be glad. I've got to start somewhere.'

'Mhmm. Start with breakfasts – does that sound to you like the best place to start?'

'And I've got to think about the snacks as well. Chocolate. Cakes. I've got a sweet tooth as well.'

'OK, take it slowly, keep it realistic, don't try and change too much all at once.'

'No, I can see that.'

John was well aware that he had moved away from a classical person-centred way of working, but he was mindful that Steve wanted to make changes and wanted to consider what was the best way to go about it. He felt that Steve was making his own decisions as to what to change, and he, John, was checking out whether it seemed realistic.

'OK, I'll tackle the breakfasts and keep an eye on the cakes.'

'Some people find it helpful to keep a record of what they eat, but not everyone's into that. Up to you.'

Keeping a record of what is being consumed can be helpful, but it's not for everyone. Care should be taken in suggesting this. The person-centred counsellor won't want to come across as if they are telling the client what's good for them, or that they are 'setting homework'. Here, the counsellor tones it down by saying that it's not for everyone. Nevertheless, a more genuinely empathic response would have been, 'mhmm, you'll focus on reducing your breakfasts and your cake intake'. This might have lead to a further discussion on the details of the changes, whereas in fact the thought of keeping a record takes the client away from this.

There is also the issue of establishing baseline measures and who introduces these, or the sharing of information relevant to a client's condition. There is no doubt that some ideas are likely to be helpful. Can they be offered by the person-centred counsellor without undermining person-centred practice (that is, undermining the process of an emerging internal locus of evaluation within the client as they free themselves from reliance on external evaluations and conditions of worth)? And if a counsellor knows something that the client is factually unaware of and which might be helpful, what does it say about the counsellor who holds back? This is surely not being transparent. There is a tension here, and there are different views. I take the view that if I have knowledge that I sense my client does not have, and which is relevant to my client's situation, then I would be open to sharing that, particularly where a client may be unknowingly and unintentionally doing damage to themselves.

Indeed, it might be argued that to not disclose potentially helpful information of this kind could be deemed unethical. My motivation would be an expression of my unconditional positive regard for my client – unconditional as it is not dependent on whether the client takes up what is offered.

Another option is for the client to obtain specific advice and information from a dietitian or nutritionist, freeing the counsellor to focus on the therapeutic work. A multi-disciplinary approach can have great value.

Steve nodded as he thought about it. It seemed like he'd be spending all day writing it down. 'Let me try what we've talked about and see how I get on.'

'Sure.'

'I know a lot of it is habit, just always eaten a lot.'

'Mhmm, that's how it has been, now it has to change.'

'Yeah. I know it.' He shook his head. 'I can't believe it, not really. I mean, you don't do you? You do what you've always done and you don't think it'll be a problem.'

'No, not a problem and then suddenly it is.'

The session continued with further discussion about Steve's eating pattern. Also his drinking was mentioned as well. It became clear that Steve quite liked a few pints some evenings.

'So, that's something else.'

'There're a lot of calories in it.'

'Yeah, and I suppose I can't switch to something too sugary, can I?'

'Best not to.'

'So much of what I do is linked to what I eat and drink, you know.'

'That's the problem, isn't it, so much linked, so many things associated with eating and drinking, and a lot of it is about what to do instead.'

'If I get bored I usually eat something.'

'Fill time?'

'Yeah, crisps, pasties, biscuits, cake, chocolate, or I'll make a sandwich. Anything really. Like I said before, I seem to spend a lot of time eating.'

'So, there's a lot to choose from in the home?'

'Well, yes there is.'

John nodded, not wanting to make any more suggestions, rather wanting to leave it with Steve to think about it.

Steve thought of the kitchen and the drawer in the sideboard with the chocolate bars in it, too much food, too much temptation. 'We've got to have less in the house. If it isn't there, well, maybe I won't eat it.'

'Mhmm, that's another strategy, cut back on what comes in.'

'Jackie likes chocolate. She's a little overweight but nothing like me. She doesn't seem to put it on like me.'

'So, Jackie has chocolate for herself, but it doesn't affect her weight too much?'

'No.' Steve paused. 'Oh shit. I came in here today angry, blaming you, pissed off, and now, well, now I'm sitting here contemplating changes that I know I've got to do, but wondering whether I can?'

'It feels uncertain. You want to make these changes, but . . .'

'You say, take it slowly, not too much at once?'

'If that feels right for you.'

'OK. I'll give it a go.'

The conversation moved on to Steve saying something about his work. He had a small business with a couple of other guys, fitting conservatories, and a little bit of window replacement. He did the estimates and some of the work, and the paperwork. The session ended with agreement for the next session to be in two weeks.

Counselling session 3: disclosures from the past

'Well, I feel I've made a start. It's not been easy, and I've not managed to change everything I want to.'

'You've made a start, Steve, and if you've begun to establish some changes then that's great. And, yeah, it's not easy.'

'No. I have had long discussions with Jackie. She's encouraging, but so long as I'm not so damned irritable. I do get irritated. I don't know why, but I just feel like I'm on a short fuse all the time.'

'Could be linked. Changing eating patterns can affect mood. Eventually, it will probably lift, but at the moment the irritations are there.'

'Yeah, I'm trying to do paperwork in the evenings and get out to the jobs more during the day. I can't just sit around at home watching TV; I end up wanting to eat something, and, well, still am most of the time. I started doing paperwork in the evening at the beginning of this week. I still go down the pub, but not every evening. Jackie and I are thinking of maybe doing other things some evenings, keep my mind off the food and the drink.'

'That makes sense. Sounds like you've been giving it a lot of thought.'

The session continued with further exploration of Steve's eating pattern, what he had changed, how he was beginning to accept less on his plate at breakfast. He'd also begun to try and reduce the sugar in his tea, but he couldn't change it in coffee, just tasted awful.

Steve again talked about how he had always eaten a lot, even as a child.

'Mhmm, so your parents were big eaters?'

'I guess so. Never went hungry. But it wasn't what I'd call excessive. My father was quite big, still is, and he eats well, but not as much as I do.'

'So, you don't think you ate particularly heavily?'

'Not early on, but later I did.'

'So, you mean you didn't eat large amounts as a child, but ate more when you grew up?'

'When I got to about twelve, thirteen.'

'Your eating pattern changed when you got to twelve or thirteen?'

Steve nodded, his thoughts going back to those years. He wondered whether to say anything about it. They weren't easy times to talk about. He didn't speak about it much, but he knew that his experiences had contributed to his decision to eat more.

'Yeah. Well, I had a tough time early on, I was kind of chubby, I guess you'd say, and got picked on a lot. Being an only child, maybe, I don't know, not having brothers, well, maybe I didn't really know how to cope. Couldn't stand up for myself much in those days, so, yeah, tough time.'

'So, your chubbiness made you a target?'

'Yeah, something like that.' He could remember the names, and he could still retreat into that small place inside himself where he wanted to just run away, but never could.

'Mhmm, so, tough time in your early childhood.' John didn't say any more in his response. He recognised that this wasn't something Steve was finding easy to talk about, so he made sure he kept himself alongside his client. His client knew what he remembered and what he felt about it, he would leave it for him to decide what he wanted to disclose, and when.

The person-centred counsellor will want to stay in contact with the client as they, in turn connect with their painful inner world. The counsellor needs to be careful and sensitive. The client is experiencing a place that may still be quite raw. The counsellor is trying to move around within, or stay in touch, with that inner world without causing disturbances or unsettling the client. Imagine the raw area to be like a damaged muscle threatening to go into spasm, too much pressure in the wrong place and it will react.

Steve nodded. 'Yeah, it was.' He sighed as he spoke. He was looking down. 'Just couldn't cope with it. So frustrated. Hated going to school. Spent a lot of time on my own, at home. Didn't really have any friends. That didn't help. No one to be with, no one to learn how to be with. Just never really had a chance at school, not then, anyway.'

'Sounds really lonely and isolated, and, as you say, no friends and on your own, and no real chance to learn the social skills you needed.'

'I was awkward as well, painfully shy, just never really coped. Used to feel sick. Hated it, hated it all.'

'Hated the whole experience, awkward, shy, not coping, feeling sick – hated it all.' John kept close to Steve's description. Steve was still staring down, clearly very much in his own inner world of experience. John simply wanted to let him know he was there, listening, but without disturbing the process.

'Just couldn't cope with it, simple as that. I had a horrible time. Fucking kids. Bastards. Made my life a fucking misery, you know?' Steve looked up and met John's eyes.

John saw the pain on Steve's face, he really had connected with that past, and it clearly made an impact on him in the present. The truth was, he didn't know. All he knew was what Steve had told him, and the sense he had from the look in Steve's eyes.

'I can't pretend to know what it was like for you, Steve, but I can see the pain in your eyes now as you talk about it.'

Steve took a deep breath, tightened his lips and tensed his jaw. 'You'd think you'd forget it, but you don't do you?'

'Not always, no.'

'I found a way, though. Classic tale, I guess, the bullied became the bully.'

'You changed from bullied to bully?'

Steve nodded. 'I had a kind of growth spurt around that age and the chubbiness kind of wore off. I was always hungry and, well, I ate more and got bigger and, well, I beat one kid up who'd been having a go. It could have been any of them, but it was him, Paul, I can see it now. I beat the shit out of him. Got into real trouble, but I got respect. And that felt good. I mean, I lost it when I went for him, blind rage, frustration, anger, I just went for it and, well, having not really hit anyone in anger like that before, I guess I hadn't appreciated my own strength. And then I knew that I was strong. And I began to get into sport, and people would back off. I'd use my size, my weight. It wasn't all fat then, you know. I could put myself about, and I did.' He shook his head. 'Crazy times, but that was how it was. And I stayed with it, football, yeah?'

'Mhmm.'

'Used to look for trouble. That's how it was. Didn't give a fuck about anyone or anything, got bevvied up and got stuck in.'

'So, a lot of violence in, what, teenage years?'

'Pretty much. But I kind of got out of it in my early twenties. Started getting serious with Jackie around then. She calmed me down quite a lot. Still got angry, always had a short fuse though better with it now.' He thought of the push on Jackie and winced inside himself. He knew he'd been out of order.

'So, Jackie calmed you down, but you've still got something of a short fuse.'

'Don't like being told what to do, I really react. Anyone who has a go at me, it's like I'll ignore it, but then I'll react. If I don't walk away, well, I have to, you know. But I guess all this weight stuff is about people telling me what to do as well, and I react to that. I know that people are saying it to help, but I react. I don't want to know. I don't want to hear.'

John nodded, 'not wanting to hear, not wanting to be told.'

'Does my head in. But that's not good enough. I know it isn't. I can't keep going round like some crazed teenager, kicking off.'

'You can't do it, but it's part of you, yeah?'

'Yeah, it's still there, still inside me. And you know, crazy thing is, there are times when I'll want to retreat as well, hide away, run away. That's not there so much, but it's around. Yeah, sometimes I want to react, kick off, stop people telling me what to do, and at other times I just want to get away. It's people laughing at me, making jokes, that kind of stuff, that's what I can't handle. Used to eat to make myself feel better. That's what I did, as a kid, I ate sweets and cakes and stuff. I sort of felt better if I felt full. Crazy really, it could only make me chubbier, but that's how it was. Doesn't make sense, does it?'

'May not now, but at the time . . .'

'. . . at the time, well, I guess it must have done.' Steve took a deep breath, nodding slightly to himself.

'So, as a child you ate to feel better, you developed a want, to escape, to run away, from being laughed at and later as you grew bigger, you found being a bully earned you respect, you ate then to grow, got into violence through football, then met Jackie, things calmed down. But you've still got that short fuse, still want to react against people telling you what to do, but still really sensitive to anyone who laughs at, or makes fun of you.'

After a series of short, empathic responses, which allowed the client to keep exploring and to talk a little more at length, the client seems to make a short comment, a sort of conclusion, and then pause. The counsellor has taken this as an opportunity to summarise what has been said. On the face of it this appears helpful, any counselling skills course would encourage this, but, this is therapeutic counselling. The client had just reached a focus in himself concerning how his eating choices in childhood made sense at the time. That has not been empathised with. A response of, 'yes, at the time it just made sense' would have held the focus and maintained the flow. The summary takes the client out of his focus, back over what has been said and leaves him potentially at least, somewhere else. His following statement reflects frustration, but is it all with himself, or could there be added frustration that his process has been diverted?

'My life history in a couple of sentences. And here I am, overweight, health at risk, having to talk to a counsellor to get my head straight.' He shook his head. 'What am I, a fucking nut case?'

'Is that how you feel?'

'Makes me wonder.'

'I want to say I hear what you say, Steve, but to me you're someone who has had to find their own way to deal with a lot of crap early in their life, and you found a way, you found ways to feel good, get respect, but, well, it's brought problems which you are now aware of and doing something about.'

'Bugger, though, isn't it?'

'Yeah.'

'I hate it when people stare at me, and they do, sometimes. Makes me feel really small inside.'

'People staring and you kind of retreat.'

'I sort of want to hide, sometimes. After a few beers, well, then I'm more likely to want to take 'em outside.' He shook his head again. 'I don't though, not these days. Did in the past. But now, well, now I try and ignore it.'

'So, a few beers and you feel, or you have felt, ready to react. Otherwise you are more likely to want to shrink inside yourself.'

'Crazy, huh?'

'I can imagine that's how it feels, but there are reasons, and that's why it isn't crazy. Few people are really crazy. Most people have reasons. You've described them to me.'

'And, you know, whilst I want to lose weight, there's a kind of nagging voice inside me that doesn't want me to, because I like being big and strong, you know. I like my size . . . and there are times when I hate it as well.'

'Yeah, like it and hate it.'

'But I've got to keep working at it, I have to, don't I?'

'Well, you know the choices, and the risks.'

'Mhmm, you have to keep working at it' would have been a more empathic response, particularly when spoken in a tone of voice reflective of, and empathic towards, how the client has spoken.

'Yeah, seen my doctor again last week. Asked me how I was doing. Told him I was seeing you and was beginning to try and reduce my eating. He was very good.

Didn't have a go. Said he thought I was doing the right thing, taking it slowly, but that I had to keep up the momentum. I guess I know that anyway, but, shit, it's hard. Feels like I'm trying to make myself go without things that I keep feeling I should have. Is that normal?'

'Like you feel you're having something taken away that you should rightfully have?'

'Yeah, I mean, I tried cutting out either the sausages or the bacon in the mornings, and I really resented it, so I have both, but less, and that's sort of easier. But looking at my plate when one or the other isn't on it, and that's what I see. It's like there's something missing that should be there. I react. I feel it, over a bloody sausage, for Christ's sake!'

'Yeah, more aware of what's missing from your plate than what's on it.'

'That's right.' He shook his head. 'Bloody weird.' He paused again. 'The fried bread was easier. I mean, I could see the sense in not having that. I have dry toast on the plate now, and that's helped me cut down on the butter. I've started having marmalade without butter as well, and we've found marmalade without sugar in the health food shop – some French make, would you believe. It's good, tastes like marmalade, actually tastes better, not so sweet but more orangey.'

'So, slowly adding to the changes?'

Steve nodded.

The session drew to a close and Steve headed off, feeling better after saying what he had during the session, and feeling somehow encouraged by the way John seemed to calmly accept all the things that he felt were so weird. There was something reassuring about how he didn't seem to look worried or concerned, just accepted it all. He didn't understand this counselling business, but maybe he didn't have to.

Points for discussion

- What particular strengths as a person-centred counsellor has John evidenced in these two sessions? How might he have been more effective?
- What were the key therapeutic moments during these sessions?
- How would you relate the content of these sessions to the processes of change described in Appendices 1 and 2?
- How have these two sessions left you feeling towards Steve? Have your feelings changed from the outset and, if so, how and why?
- What might have been different in these sessions had the counsellor been female and small? What different issues might have arisen for the counsellor and the client?
- What would you be taking to supervision from these sessions if you were the counsellor?
- Write notes for these two sessions.

CHAPTER 3

Progress so far . . .

The next few sessions have seen Steve continue to focus on the changes to his eating. He has had a few lapses, usually at times when he was feeling frustrated and wanting something to make him feel good. He recognised how he still used food as a comforter. It also came to light that he used it to sometimes react against his wife. It would provoke her and there were times when that was what he wanted to do, particularly if she had had a go because he'd eaten more than he'd said he would, or had a few extra beers in the evening. 'She wanted to moan, he'd give her something to moan about.' They explored it in the counselling session. Steve admitted that it wasn't really a very helpful reaction, that he needed to deal with things in a different way.

Generally, though, Jackie was supportive, and that was proving helpful. John had wondered whether Steve might want her to come along for a session; clients sometimes asked if their partner could attend, to get a feel for what was happening, help them to understand, particularly where it was proving a difficult process. But Steve hadn't suggested this and John wasn't going to. It was Steve's time and maybe he wanted to keep it that way.

Steve had had six sessions and the weight was coming off, and pretty much in line with national guidelines. Three months he had been attending the counselling and he had lost just over a stone. The national guidelines recommend a weight loss of 1 lb per week, or 5 per cent weight loss in 12 weeks, which for Steve would amount to about 13 lb. Steve had reduced a little faster than this. He was aiming for the twenty-stone barrier, that was his first target. John felt confident he would make it. He seemed very motivated. Steve had also started to take more exercise, slowly and with agreement from his GP. He was going out for walks more, trying to at least get into a routine of taking exercise.

Counselling session 7: sadness, and a 'hole full of emptiness' is encountered

'It's coming down. I've got one of those pedometers; little thing you attach to your belt. I'm measuring how far I walk. It's amazing how much you do just walking around, but I'm trying to make sure I walk the best part of three to four miles a day, counting everything, and I'm managing it quite easily, and days when we deliberately go on a walk, well, it's easily over that. And I'm beginning to feel different. I know I've still got a long way to go, but I do feel different.' Steve was genuinely pleased with his progress, and his weight was still coming down. Both he and Jackie were now working together at a totally different lifestyle. But in spite of everything, it still wasn't easy. The urges for a bacon sandwich when he knew he wasn't actually hungry, remained a huge temptation and, yes, he had weakened occasionally. And he said to himself it was just a one-off, and he knew as well he was kind of rewarding himself a bit as well, for doing so well. And it generally was a one-off, but it happened and he knew he had to feel more in control.

Generally, though, his diet had improved. Less fat, less sugar, more whole-food. But he was also aware that his moods still fluctuated a lot. It felt as though his whole system was trying to adjust to the changes he was making. He still got irritated and frustrated very easily. He would have phases of poor concentration. Some days everything just seemed too much of an effort. But, like he said, he generally felt an improvement, but he was aware of these fluctuations.

'So, feeling different, good different?'

'Mainly, but those mood shifts I mentioned before, they're still happening. But it's like they come and go – can't be sure when, though. But in general, I do feel better for it. But I know I'm not very easy to get on with some days.'

'So your mood affects how you are with other people?'

'I can get moody and withdrawn. I guess it's part of the process.'

'You're making lots of changes to your life, to yourself.'

'I know, but I also know I need to do more.'

'Mhmm, that sense of needing to do more.'

'I know I have to lose more weight, but I suppose I have to be patient.' He grimaced.

'You don't sound as though that's too easy.'

The counsellor is empathising perhaps more to the way the client has spoken, and to the expression on his face, than to what has been said. Empathy is not only about conveying what is received from verbal communication. We are a very verbal culture in terms of communication, but a person uses voice tones and facial expressions and other body language to express what they think and feel. The person-centred counsellor will want to receive this as well, and demonstrate their empathy for what has been communicated to them.

However, to simply focus on body language or voice tone can be invasive for the client. Often thoughts and feelings are communicated in this way without the client being aware of them. Too much of this kind of empathy, particularly early on in a therapeutic relationship, can leave the client feeling stripped naked psychologically or emotionally, leaving them self-conscious and over-sensitive as they try to control what they communicate.

> Bear in mind that a client attends for counselling because they are to some degree in a state of incongruence. They may be anxiously trying to contain something. The counsellor wants the client to feel able to express themselves freely. Having a sense that the counsellor is studying you and waiting to pick up on every little detail of which you are unaware can be anxiety provoking and is not an experience of person-centred counselling.

'No, it isn't. I mean, I really wonder just how far I should go with this as well. I wonder sometimes about when to stop. I mean, eighteen stone, sixteen, fourteen? I can't see myself managing more than that, and maybe I won't get that far anyway. I mean, it's been over three months already. I'm under twenty-one stone now and aiming for twenty.'

'How far do you want to go, Steve?' John wanted Steve to really connect with his own thoughts and feelings on this.

'I guess when I think about it, I don't know. I mean, I don't want to be thin – hard to imagine, I know, but, well, I do want to keep some weight.'

'Some weight is important to you to keep, yes?'

'Well, yes, it is. I can't imagine being me and not having weight, you know, it, well, it sort of seems unreal somehow.'

'Trying to imagine yourself with a lot less weight, it's just not something you can do.'

'I'm used to how I feel. My size is important to me.'

'Mhmm. It's – and sorry for the pun but it's a big part of you.'

Steve smiled. There wasn't really any other way of saying it. 'Nice one, yes, I know. It is. It is so much who I am.'

'Who you are.'

Steve nodded. 'I suppose my size has been a major factor in shaping me, the person, me, Steve, you know?' He went quiet, the words 'fat bastard' had come to mind; he'd been called that a few times. On a good day, he laughed, brushed it off, he could even make a joke of it himself, though if he was really honest with himself he would have to admit that at some level it hurt. On a bad day? Two reactions. Want to get away, hideaway, though that happened less rarely. More often he'd want to punch the lights out of whoever had said it.

John did not appreciate what Steve was thinking, he simply heard what he had said and noted the silence that had followed. 'Yeah, a big part in you being the person that you are.' He knew that the humour of a few minutes ago had passed, the atmosphere had changed. Steve was in another place. He spoke the words with greater seriousness and with a flatter tone.

> The counsellor must be ready for moods and atmospheres to change rapidly within the therapeutic relationship. Humour one moment, sadness or seriousness the next. The counsellor's tone of voice, as much as what they say, will convey their empathy for these shifts that necessarily occur.

The silence continued. John sensed that Steve seemed suddenly quite withdrawn in some way. The silence felt to him as though it was difficult, sad, not awkward though. He felt suddenly tired as he sat there, seeking to maintain his attention on Steve. Suddenly he felt incredibly tired. He wanted to yawn. Should I stifle it, he wondered, but he knew that there was little point. Yet he hadn't felt tired . . . He yawned.

Steve was still looking down. He'd sensed a movement but not what was happening for John. He remained locked in his own thoughts about himself. He felt heavy, weighed down. It was like something had suddenly switched or changed inside himself. He sighed without realising that he had sighed. And he was shaking his head ever so slightly, though again unaware of this movement.

John noted the slight shaking of Steve's head. Was it an intentional communication, or something emerging from within Steve that he was reacting to and unintentionally expressing it through that movement? He guessed the latter. He knew that whilst there might be some justification in acknowledging the movement in a situation of very minimal contact – in a pre-therapy situation – that was certainly not the case here. It would be much more likely to jolt Steve away from what he was experiencing, making him suddenly aware of something that, in the moment, was probably outside of his awareness.

Steve continued to sit. It felt as though he didn't want to move, didn't want to do anything. Yes, that heaviness was there, but not a physical heaviness. He was used to that. There was something else and he felt like it was gluing him down. And yet, at the same time, it wasn't as if he was really thinking about it or analysing it; that was simply how it was. He was somehow glued down inside himself. He suddenly felt quite sad, the feeling bubbling up from nowhere. It took him totally by surprise. He tried to contain it, but it wasn't going to be contained. It felt as though it suddenly filled his whole being. His throat felt like a lump had appeared in it from nowhere. And his stomach suddenly felt empty, hollow, it was a strange feeling and yet somehow familiar. But it was the sadness. He felt his eyes watering. But he didn't know what he was sad about, but it was there . . .

Steve didn't finish his thoughts, and it had all happened very quickly. Now tears were flowing out of his eyes, he could feel them on his cheeks. He swallowed hard, trying to stem the flow, but he couldn't. It was like a bubble of tears had suddenly burst somewhere behind his eyes and they just poured out. He felt embarrassed. He didn't like to cry, and not in front of another man. He didn't know what to do, how to react, and he couldn't think about that because of the sadness that rose up inside him. At least, it emerged but was more of a bubble bursting again, and once burst there was no way to contain it.

John looked on, watching Steve's shoulders rise and fall as the tears flowed from his eyes. Steve had now lifted his right hand and was pinching his eyes either side of his nose. The tears continued to escape. His breath came in short gasps. His throat was burning, his chest felt as though it was being pressed upon, as if it was hard to expand it. He swallowed again, the tears continued, the feelings persisted. Sadness, and suddenly such emptiness, he felt so deeply empty inside. He wasn't trying to find words, this was simply his experience. As though inside his skin he didn't exist, and yet he did, he hurt so much. He was very present and yet so empty, so, so empty.

John sat, wondering if he should offer Steve a tissue, or say something, but he genuinely felt that to do so would be to maybe take Steve's focus away, and it felt to him that whatever he was experiencing – and releasing – needed to come out. He needed to trust the process that was causing so many tears and, quite clearly, so much distress. He didn't want to say or do anything that might disturb what was happening, so he remained attentive, aware that his senses were suddenly so much more alert. The tiredness that had crept into him just before had passed.

An interesting dilemma. Offering a tissue would seem a very natural thing to do, and at times will be quite appropriate in a situation like this, however, there are occasions when it is right to let the client remain with what they are experiencing and not risk distracting them. Offering a tissue can be taken as a sign that it's time to stop the tears. When in doubt, let the process continue, and if the counsellor says something to remind the client of their presence – and generally the client is well aware of the counsellor, unless they have slipped into a deeper, more traumatised region – then it should be done quietly, gently, so as not to disturb the process and focus within the client. And, of course, feelings of warmth and unconditional positive regard should be maintained within the heart of the counsellor.

Steve opened his mouth to say something but he couldn't get any words out. He wanted to apologise, but the sadness, the feelings inside him were so raw, and he could only continue breathing in small breaths, interspersed with swallows. It continued, he tried again to control it, tried to tighten his closed eyes a little more, but that made no difference, his breathing switched to his nose and to a succession of very short in-breaths and out-breaths which were not breaths at all, just air passing in and out of his nose with each sob, his mouth closed tight, no air passing into his lungs.

'Oh God.' He eventually managed to say, and this was immediately lost in a further series of sobs, his shoulders rising and falling in, what seemed to John, to be painful and wracking movements.

John decided that as Steve had managed to speak he should now respond. 'Stay with it, Steve, it's OK, you're letting it out, letting it go.'

Steve, still with his eyes closed shut, still pinching into the corner of his eyes with his right thumb and forefinger, nodded, swallowed, opened his mouth and breathed in, trying to acknowledge John, but his mouth closed again as another wave of emotion hit him. He hadn't realised how much he had been clenching his left fist. Only now he began to realise how much tension he had in his left arm, running up into his shoulder and his left breast. He'd never, ever, felt anything like this before. Yes, he knew he'd been sad and lonely at times in the past, but nothing like this.

Steve made a final superlative effort to get control, a final tightening of his lips and of his closed eyes, a swallow and a deep breath and he lifted up his head, opened his eyes and blew out a short breath, swallowed again, and took another deep breath, again blowing it out through his mouth. He felt wretched, absolutely wretched. He swallowed again, his throat felt raw, the lump wouldn't move. He felt a yawn coming on, he couldn't stifle it. His eyes felt raw as well, and still very watery. His cheeks and the collar of his shirt against his neck felt wet.

He looked at John and caught the expression on John's face. He looked – he didn't know what word to use – but he seemed to be there, seemed to be somehow there, he didn't have words for it. But it felt somehow good, and he felt embarrassed as well. That was it, somehow he looked so accepting. Yes, he looked concerned, but there was a warmth, a caring, a compassion – was that what it was? – in his eyes. He saw John tighten his lips and nod his head slightly. It was an acknowledgement where there was nothing to say. Steve didn't know what he wanted or expected John to say, and somehow it didn't matter, John was there. He wasn't alone with what he had experienced although at the time he had felt utterly . . . He took a deep breath again.

'Ohh God.' He shook his head. Another breath which he blew out, still shaking his head. His back was aching – it often did, but just at the moment he was very aware of it. He moved his arms and his shoulders back to try and free the discomfort, shifted from side to side as well, trying to unlock the tension that had built up. It triggered another yawn. He suddenly felt very tired, absolutely drained. 'What – what was that?'

'Something, I think, that you have been carrying around for a long time.'

'I never realised, I never knew, I mean, I felt so utterly out-of-control, I couldn't do anything. So much emotion. So much . . .' He shook his head. The word 'sadness' was in his head but somehow he felt a reluctance to say it. He wasn't sure if it would trigger another emotional reaction.

'Yeah, lots and lots of emotion, and . . .' John also left his sentence unfinished, acknowledging that Steve had not finished what he had said and leaving it open for him to say more if he wanted to.

Steve looked at John and swallowed. He had to say it. 'Sadness.' He said it quietly, and very reflectively, as though it was something given to him that he had to handle very carefully. He blinked as he said it.

John nodded, and replied in a similarly quiet tone. 'Sadness, lots and lots of sadness.'

Steve's turn to nod. He was taking another deep breath, feeling the air filling his lungs. His throat burned a little less now, the lump was subsiding.

'It was suddenly there, like . . . , like . . . , I don't know, it was inside me and it just burst. Just suddenly, there it was, bang and that was it.'

'Like an explosion inside yourself?' John was responding to the bang, seeking to empathise with what Steve was describing.

Steve frowned. 'No, not an explosion, not like that, not like a . . . , I don't know, more like a balloon bursting, but that's not right either.'

'So, not an explosion, something like a balloon bursting but different to that.' John had the thought of wondering how they'd got into describing the sensation rather than describing the emotions, but maybe that was what Steve needed as he re-orientated and adjusted from his experience. He hoped he hadn't directed him, but he couldn't think what he had said and besides there wasn't time for that. He had to stay with Steve, with his focus.

'I remember going quiet, really quiet. I don't mean not saying anything, but it was like I went really quiet inside, you know?'

John nodded.

'And I felt, yes, I remember feeling kind of stuck, glued down, sort of heavy but in a strange kind of way.'

John nodded again, 'heavy and stuck down, but it was a strange kind of heavy and stuckness?'

Steve nodded, 'and then, then I just suddenly felt so sad.' The lump was back in his throat and his eyes were watering again.

'So sad?'

Steve had closed his eyes as John was responding, he could feel the emotions again, but nothing like before, these were far more manageable. 'I feel so sad, and so empty.'

John noted the switch into the present tense.

Whereas before Steve was so caught up in the experience and unable to communicate his experience in words, now that he is re-experiencing it but in a less intense manner, he is able to describe what he is feeling. He has not been pressured into describing them, he has conveyed what the process felt like and now he is in a place to be able to describe the emotional landscape, as it were, that is – the nature of the emotions that he has suddenly encountered.

'So sad and empty.' John spoke softly, not wanting his empathic response to intrude on Steve's experience, not wanting his voice to be a distraction that might in effect pull Steve's focus out of what was present within his own inner world of experience.

Steve heard John and the words seemed to slide by. He remained feeling sad, and the emptiness, he realised, had left him ravenously hungry. He swallowed and opened his eyes again. 'It's still very close.'

'And may be for a while.'

Steve was shaking his head, looking mystified, at least that was how it was striking John. 'Something puzzling you?'

'I just feel so incredibly hungry. I mean, really, really hungry.'

'Mhmm. Suddenly you want to eat?'

'I do, but, well, I don't. It's like, I feel really hungry and yet I'm also thinking that I don't want to eat, and both at the same time.'

'So you don't want to eat but you are feeling incredibly hungry.'

Steve remained puzzled, but he wanted to make sense of it. He'd just come through something that was unlike anything he'd ever experienced, and survived, he was still breathing, still in one piece, and he wanted to make sense of what had happened and was happening.

'I . . . , yeah, I mean I do want to eat, and I don't.'

'Mhmm, that experience has left you wanting to eat and not wanting to eat.'

'It's like . . . , I don't know, I can't describe it, but it's like I feel so empty, I just want to fill myself up.'

'Fill up that emptiness inside yourself.'

Steve was taking a deep breath, aware that his stomach felt hollow, but it was more than his stomach, there just felt like a real emptiness in that part of his body, and it extended up towards his chest. It was weird.

Steve heard himself say something which stopped his thinking for a moment. 'It won't fill me, though.' The words were spoken quite quietly.

'It won't fill you?' Again, John matched the volume and tone of what Steve had said.

Steve was shaking his head. 'No, it won't, it never did, and it still won't.'

John stayed focused on Steve and what he was saying, listening intently, feeling it was suddenly particularly important that Steve experienced being heard, received and accepted.

'Something never did fill you and never will?'

Steve nodded, and having been looking away he now looked back at John. 'I would eat to feel comfortable, to feel, I don't know, to feel full. I liked the feeling, I liked the sensation. I felt somehow better if I had a full stomach, I don't know, that sensation, that's what I did. I mean, that's how I coped when I was a kid. I used to eat to feel full. But what I'm now wondering. No, not wondering, I know, I was eating to fill . . .' Steve paused. A word had come to mind that he hadn't really thought about before. 'It was like filling a hole, a huge hole. And you know, and this is going to sound really weird. But the hole, I mean, how can I say it?' He paused.

'Try and say it as it is, we can make sense of the words later.'

That sounded a good response. 'It's like a hole that's full of emptiness.' Steve took a deep breath. There was something about having said it in that way. A kind of relief. A sort of, yes, that's it, I've named it, I've made it visible.

'A hole that's full of emptiness.' John empathised using Steve's words, aware that whilst he could attach a meaning to the words that he used, exactly what Steve's experience was he did not know. He guessed that the expression on his face would have a searching tone to it.

'It's not easy to make sense of, and yet . . . ,'

'To you it makes perfect sense, the idea of a hole, a place where there is nothing yet it is full.'

'Emptiness is not nothing.'

'No, and that's the key.'

'I felt a lot of emptiness, and that made me sad, and I ate to feel better, to fill the emptiness, to make the sadness go away.'

John nodded. These were profound recognitions and he so appreciated the emotional literacy that Steve had. He really wanted to try and make sense of what he had experienced, or so it seemed.

The session began to wind down. Steve was tired, so was John. It felt as though somehow, for the moment, there was little more to say. A profound experience had occurred and Steve knew something had shifted, had changed inside him. He needed time to make sense of it. And he was still aware of that hunger. They discussed it and looked at ways to try and avoid eating on that feeling. Steve could see that logically, it wasn't really hunger, not physical hunger anyway. Steve concluded that perhaps he needed to not try and cut anything else out until this feeling passed. That maybe he should stabilise, though if he felt able to eat less at any time then to do so. He wasn't sure how he was going to be. He didn't want things to get away from him.

John asked him what might help and Steve replied that maybe he needed to see him weekly, just for a bit. Somehow two weeks suddenly seemed like a long time.

John agreed to this, thinking that perhaps Steve's internal experience had perhaps left him sensitive to any feelings of facing something on his own. They agreed an appointment for the next week.

After the session John found himself pondering on the nature of empathy. What was it? He knew what he read in the books, and the debates about whether it was right to talk about empathy or empathic understanding, or whether understanding was the right term because maybe understanding required a direct experience of that which the client experienced and so maybe appreciation was a better word to use. But it was another issue that was in his mind, and it was about what aspect of the empathic experience was of most therapeutic significance. Was it the actual act of listening and hearing the client as they spoke or communicated what they needed to communicate by some other means, or was it the responding by the counsellor after the client had finished their communication that mattered most? Of course, the two were bound together, but it seemed to John that maybe what was most important was the client's sense of being heard, listened to, understood *as they were speaking* that was most significant. The response from the counsellor was merely a kind of confirmation. It left him more aware of the need to really be attentive to the client, that perhaps it was in those periods when he was listening to the client, and his face was conveying his human reactions to what was being said; his warmth, his acceptance, a look of understanding in his eyes, maybe, perhaps those were the times that mattered most and not the verbal element of his attending to his client that followed. That had to be there, yes, but you do not need someone telling you what you have just said to feel heard. It's an instinct, an inner knowing, and that was surely what was important to bear in mind when thinking about how empathy or empathic understanding is communicated. A thought sprang to mind, an 'ah-ha moment': is empathy what is communicated when the client speaks, and empathic understanding what is communicated verbally when the client stops speaking?

Points for discussion

- How did John communicate his empathy and acceptance to Steve?
- What were the facilitative moments in this session?
- How did you feel as you read this session? Had you been John, what would you have found most challenging or difficult?
- Would you have responded at any time in a different way to Steve? Why and what is your theoretical reason for this?
- How does Steve's experience relate to Rogers' seven stages of change?
- What are your reactions to the final paragraph above?
- Write notes for this session.

CHAPTER 4

Supervision

'I've talked about Steve before.'

Chloe nodded. She'd been struck by how well he had been doing, and how he was engaging in the process, accepting that his work at reducing his weight was only part of the process.

'Mhmm, so, you want to bring me up-to-date?'

'Yes. I saw him earlier this week and, well, he really did connect with some feelings.'

'New feelings?'

'Feelings that were new to him in a sense, though emerging from his past.'

'So, feelings from the past, and feelings relevant to his process?'

'Very much so. I think they emerged because of the process of change that Steve has been going through.'

'So the loosening process is having an impact, then?'

'Seems to be, and I guess I was left pondering on Rogers' stages of change, how the bubbling up of feelings is equated with stage six. I'm not sure how linear that process is.'

'You mean people jump around between the stages?'

'More that I think people can be at different stages with different issues, although there is also a general movement as well towards more fluidity, but not every-thing is loosened at the same time – thank goodness.'

Chloe nodded. 'Quite, I don't know that people would be able to cope with all the blocked up feelings emerging at the same time, though they can cluster.'

'Well, he described it, I thought, really vividly. Something like how it burst inside him, but not like something going bang.'

'More like a bubble than a balloon, the containing skin is somehow very thin and tears rather than bursts.'

'He didn't describe it like that but hearing you say that, well, yes, maybe.'

'Well, it may not be his experience. But you say he definitely had this sense of feelings emerging and bursting open inside him.' Chloe was aware of not yet knowing quite what the feelings were, but she knew that John would get around to that.

'And there was such a powerful release of emotion, a really powerful moment well, more than a moment, it went on for some time.'

'Mhmm. And how did you receive it?' Chloe wanted to check John's responsiveness to what was occurring.

'I felt very still, actually. I was aware of thinking that I really couldn't risk disturbing what was happening for Steve. It's like, do I remind him I'm there, or make some comment about what is happening? But I decided not to, I didn't want to say or do anything that would take his attention away from what was happening inside of him.'

'I think that's very wise, and I also think that sometimes, when these really deep emotions emerge, we wouldn't be able to distract them anyway. What is being experienced is too present, too overwhelming for a comment from us to take them out of it. But, best to play safe and trust the process.'

'So, I sat quietly but holding my attention very much on Steve, trying to be fully available, to be sensitive to what was happening. I really believe that's important. I know the client may not see you in those moments – Steve had his eyes closed, his hands to his face, his head lowered, but I feel that there is something that gets communicated even though there are no apparent physical means for that to be received.'

'As if the client, at some level, or in some subjective way, is aware of your presence even though he cannot see or hear you?'

'More than that, as if he knows or can maybe sense, and maybe not consciously, but there is a knowing that there is a person in the room who is listening and being with you in spirit, I think that's what I mean – being there in spirit.'

'So, a sense of having someone being there in spirit.'

'And maybe that's something that the client has already developed from their experience of being with their counsellor. So, I mean, Steve has already sat with me for however many sessions it was – six or seven – he knows whether I am attentive, whether I am there in spirit with him. And maybe if he has had that experience enough times he starts to carry an assumption that I still will be attentive even when he is so engrossed in his own emotional release that he may be barely aware of my presence.' John stopped to ponder what he had said. He continued before Chloe had a chance to respond. 'But of course, the very emotional release may bring with it a whole range of associated thoughts and feelings that could cast doubt on whether anyone could be there for him.' He paused again. 'I don't know, I just think that being attentive even if there is no apparent way that that is being communicated, is important.'

'Like holding a respectful attitude for your client?'

'That's part of it, yes, respecting their need to be as they are. It's not that I want to be voyeuristic or anything like that. I'm not sitting with some morbid fascination. I simply want to sit with a sense of being with my client, being a presence, a person, a someone sharing ... That's not quite right, I think I need to create my own vocabulary here.'

'Go on.'

'It's like I'm sort of sharing Steve's experience although of course I'm not, I'm only witnessing the physical reactions to what he is experiencing inside, and my thoughts and feelings in response to that. But I want to say something like I feel "shared into" the experience, but I'm not quite sure what I mean by that.'

'Shared into?'

John paused. What did he mean? When he first thought of those words they felt right. Having heard himself say them, and hearing Chloe repeat them back, he wondered, what did he mean? What was he trying to get at?

'You know, it's like if you share something with someone, let's say a piece of apple pie, let's say we share a pie here. You have a piece and I have a piece. We remain separate in the room, you there, me here, and we each have our own separate pieces of pie although they come from the same pie and we are probably both tasting the same things when we eat it, although I'll have my associations with the experience of eating apple pie, and you'll have yours. But whilst there is a shared experience, in fact we are separate in our experiencing. Does that make sense?'

'Mhmm, I think so. We are separate within the shared experience of eating the pie. The pie and the fact that we are both eating it is the shared experience, everything else is separate and individual to each of us.'

John nodded. 'OK, so when I say "shared into" the experience, what am I saying?' He paused, 'it's like, yes, let's go back to the pie, though it may lose something because I think it's quite subtle. But it's like as I eat my piece of pie I am also observing your experience of eating your piece of pie and am in some way therefore being shared into your experience. We share the pie, but it becomes shared into when I am in some way bringing into myself an awareness of your experience.'

'OK, I can see that, you get a sense of my pie-eating experience.'

'So where does that leave me?' John thought about it again. 'Yes, so, yes, I cannot share Steve's experience, but by being attentive to how he is, how he looks, how his body is, the sounds he's making, then I can be "shared into" his experience.' John shook his head, that didn't seem right. Didn't seem to capture quite what he meant. It still had a tone of separateness to it. He wanted to capture a sense of some kind of merging. Yes, that was the word. 'It's like a kind of merging takes place, or at least, that's what I am seeking to achieve. A merging, trying to raise my sensitivity in some way so that I can get under the outer appearance.' He looked at Chloe. 'Am I making any sense here, or am I just tangling myself up in a knot?'

'Is that how it feels?'

'A bit.'

'Well, what I am hearing is you trying to find the words that feel right for you to explain your striving to get behind the appearance, get behind the sights and the sounds, to achieve some kind of merging at some subtler level, and that merging is something about being "shared into" your client's experience'. Chloe raised her eyebrows. 'Am I catching it?'

John nodded. 'Yes. Yes. So it is about trying to open myself to what Steve is experiencing more than what he is expressing.'

'OK, that's clear. But my thought to that is, how can you do that? What mechanism is there for that to occur? We are reliant on what comes through our senses. And we then attach meanings to those experiences. But they are reactions to what our client shows us, not what is actually happening inside him, or her.'

'I just get a sense that there is something more. I don't know, we seem so bound up by the physical senses, you know, but what about atmospheres? You go into a room and you feel something. You don't know what it is, or why, but it's there. Is it us producing that as a response to the stimulus of the shape, colour, whatever of the room, or can we sense more?'

'Can we sense the unseen?'

'Yes, yes, and that's it, that's it exactly, can we sense the unseen and, if we can, how can we work with that?'

Chloe nodded. She wasn't sure she fully agreed with what John was saying, but she did accept his experience and his questioning. She knew people did believe that we could communicate in ways other than through physical means – telepathy, for instance. She wasn't convinced, herself, but she wasn't going to condemn the idea. She didn't know. She'd had experiences herself that had left her wondering. Thinking of someone just as they phoned her, particularly someone that she hadn't seen or thought about for some time. That was kind of spooky, but maybe those things happened, it was chance but it had special meaning placed on it when it occasionally happened.

'So, working with the idea that we can connect with our clients in some deeper, more immediate way, as if we literally do enter their world. I mean, not a matter of imagining it, or of responding only to what the client tells us, but to actually be in it in some way?'

'That's what I mean. And so that's the attitude I want to be open to. I can't make myself go into the unseen, but it feels as though it is important to be open to the possibility of that kind of connection.'

'So, holding the possibility in mind?'

'And being attentive to what comes into my awareness in those moments because it may have particular significance.'

'You saying that reminds me of that comment by Rogers about when he felt himself in a slightly altered state of consciousness, how did the passage go ...' Chloe glanced over to her bookshelves. She got up and took *A Way of Being* off the shelf. She flicked through the pages. 'Yes, here we are: "I find that when I am closest to my inner, intuitive self ..." I wonder what he meant by that? Never mind, " when I am somehow in touch with the unknown in me, when perhaps I am in a slightly altered state of consciousness, then whatever I do seems to be full of healing. Then simply my *presence* is releasing and helpful to the other". And he goes on to say about acting in ways that he can't justify logically, but they seem to be helpful. And then, yes, this bit. "It seems that my inner spirit has reached out and touched the inner spirit of the other. Our relationship transcends itself and becomes a part of something larger. Profound growth and healing energy are present" (Rogers, 1980, p. 129). Is this the sort of thing you are getting at?'

'In a way, yes, but I think whereas Rogers was describing something that spontaneously can happen in moments of deep contact, when there is a merging in some way, I think what I'm saying is that I think in silences in particular, or when a client is undergoing intense emotional release, we try to be open to the possibility of that merging, and yes, something about *presence* as well.

Something about ..., maybe it's about being open to being "shared into" my client's world of experience and in that process there is something important about *presence*. There's something else he wrote in there.' John pointed to the book in Chloe's hand.

Chloe passed him the book.

'I'm not sure if I can find it, but it is a section in which he talks about modern physics, mystical experiences, Carlos Castaneda, Lawrence LeShan, and I think it was Fritjof Capra. Let me see if I can find it.'

It was John's turn to flick through the book. 'Yes, here we are, page 256. Yes, he writes openly about possibilities for experiencing beyond the five senses, but this bit, here: "Perhaps in the coming generations of younger psychologists, hopefully unencumbered by the university prohibitions and resistances, there will be a few who will dare to investigate the possibility that there is a lawful reality which is not open to our five senses; a reality in which present, past, and future are intermingled, in which space is not a barrier, and time has disappeared; a reality which can be perceived and known only when we are passively receptive, rather than actively bent on knowing. This is one of the most exciting challenges posed to psychology" (Rogers, 1980, p. 256). So, what do we make of that?'

'He was looking beyond the five senses to make sense of experiences that people testify to.'

'The bit about being "passively receptive", that's what I think it's about, and that's what I was trying to be, open to, I don't know, a something, a touch of my client's inner world.'

'A direct apprehension of the truth of his experience, unaffected by expression.' Chloe hadn't really thought about what she was going to say, the words just came together.

'That sounds good.'

'Mhmm, OK. So, I'm going to acknowledge the importance of all that we have been discussing here, and bring it back to you and to Steve.'

'But that's it, trying to get a direct sense of his experience without him having to tell me what it is.'

'To be directly touched by his emotion in some way?'

'Why not?'

'OK, but we still have no mechanism for it, unless we accept the notion of a reality beyond the five senses which we can access somehow.'

'Yeah. And something that makes me reflect on this is the experience clients have, and I've known I've had, when a feeling does bubble up or emerge out of the past. It feels so in the present, and it comes from nowhere but feels everywhere. And I just wonder if it emerges from some other reality within us, I don't know, some dimension where feelings get locked up, you know?'

'Maybe, maybe. We can't know. At best, it is an hypothesis.'

'So, for Steve it was sadness, that was the first word he used, and then he talked about emptiness. And that emptiness made him feel hungry, and we explored that. That feels important, like he's trying to fill up his emptiness with food.'

'Emptiness from his past that he's sort of carried with him, unknowingly, or rather, without really being aware that that was what was happening.'

'Something like that. And it left him feeling really concerned that he was going to relapse on his altered eating pattern. So we agreed to weekly appointments. I think that was right. He was clearly concerned, not wanting to go back to how it was, but very aware of how he was feeling inside himself.'

'It seems quite important that he was offered that.'

'I think he suggested it, I can't remember, but it was certainly a mutual decision.'

'So, he's out there with a powerful urge to eat to fill that emptiness.'

'And my sense is that something significant has emerged and that there is more to this, more to what his emptiness means. I'm not convinced it's as simple as "eating on emptiness", but I think it is a significant component, particularly because as a child he ate to feel comfortable during the time when he was being bullied. The perverse thing – maybe that's not a good word, maybe I should say paradoxical – was that he was bullied for being chubby yet he was eating to feel full which he associated with feeling better. Something like that, anyway.'

'That's how it can be, as we know.'

John nodded.

'So, what next with Steve?'

'Well, I hope to see him next week and, well, it will be up to him what he brings to the session. I suppose he may describe how he has got on, he may want to discuss ideas to ensure he can stabilise his new eating pattern if it is still under threat. Or he might want to explore what this emptiness means to him.' He paused. 'You know, this emptiness, emotional, psychological, it's a really good example of how an external behaviour and an internal psychological process can be linked. I know it's not as simple as eating to fill a psychological void, but there is an element of this within the complexity of it all. I just think it is fascinating how internal and external processes and behaviours interact with each other, and sustainable change means changes in both.'

'Yes, both together, just the psychological and just the behavioural may make inroads, and may be enough for some people, but for others there needs to be a place for both to be addressed.'

'I feel privileged to be working in this area. I think it opens up some fascinating ideas for how psychology and behaviour are linked, and how the therapeutic climate that the person-centred approach offers can help clients to really work at depth with themselves.'

'And, once again, as we know, someone struggling in the present because of relational problems in the past. Time and again it comes back to relationship and how people internalise the experience, the introjects that they take on board through which they define themselves, who they are and what they can expect.'

John enjoyed his work. What was interesting for him was that he not only saw psychological and emotional changes in his clients, and shifts in his relational experience with them, he also saw physical changes as well. It was like an outer symbol of the inner changes taking place. But always, always, he held in mind the word 'sustainable'.

The supervision session moved on, John feeling satisfied with his exploration of his work with Steve, and of the meaning of his idea about being 'shared into' his client's experience. He thought he might write down some of these ideas, maybe it would make the basis of a paper sometime in the future.

Counselling session 8: the 'hole full of emptiness' explored

'I'm glad to see you again, John, it's been hard going. So many thoughts and feelings have been around. I've really felt so, I don't know, sensitive I guess this past week.'

'So what happened last time left you more sensitive to, what, your feelings, thoughts?'

Steve nodded. 'I'm just aware that, well, suddenly my eating is no longer just about eating. It's like everything has become something else, or at least, more than what it was.'

'More than just about how much and what you eat?'

'It's about what I do to make myself feel good. I mean, this week, I've really been aware of the urge to eat more, to start eating things that I had given up, you know? Junk food. I just suddenly get these really powerful urges to eat burgers and chips, the stuff I've really been getting away from and feeling good about avoiding. But I've really been craving it. And bread – white bread – and biscuits, you know. I keep hearing myself giving myself reasons why it's OK to have something. And I know there's no justification for it, I know it, but it's there, nagging at me.' Steve shook his head and took a deep breath.

'So, it's been a bloody hard week, trying to cope with the cravings.'

'I thought that maybe after last week I'd feel different, once I sort of got over it. But it's left me somehow wanting to eat more. I don't know. I mean, it's not as though I've been feeling like I did last week, I mean, not all the time. Sometimes, sometimes I've felt it.' He lapsed into silence, aware of how close the feelings were.

'So you have continued to feel like you did last week some of the time, and it leaves you wanting to eat more.'

'And I know that I can't, I mustn't. And, yes, OK, I have slipped up a couple of times. I know I have. I had a burger and chips I didn't need last Friday, and again on Monday. I guess I had nothing around me to stop me. Driving back from a job late afternoon.' He took a deep breath and sighed. 'Is it always going to be like this?'

John shook his head. 'What's happened has put you in touch with a really sensitive part of yourself, and it's very connected to your urge to eat.'

The counsellor has offered an explanation. He hasn't answered the question. It is not an empathic response. However, the explanation has emerged out of the counsellor's feeling of connection towards the client and it does convey meaning to the client whose reaction is immediate. It is perhaps an example of the counsellor observing, if you like, the client's inner world and seeing something that the client hasn't yet seen, but the moment he points it out the client is able to affirm it for himself. Nevertheless, it was an explanation and not an empathic response, and did not answer the question or reflect the client's need to ask the question. The client is left not knowing the answer to 'is it always going to be like this?'.

'Too bloody right. And you know, I find myself thinking about it, but that can just make it worse. It's like I want to think about it to make sense of it, but when I do I just end up feeling that craving for food. It's a fucking nightmare, it really is. I mean, I don't know. I didn't think it would suddenly be this hard.'

'Comes as a shock.'

'It's so powerful. It's thinking about it. If I didn't do that, maybe it would be easier, but I have to, I need to make sense of it, I need to know I can make other choices. And at the moment I feel like I'm slipping back. I don't know if I can do it.' Steve looked so distraught as he finished what he was saying. It wasn't surprising, he really was wondering whether he could sustain his change of diet and eating pattern. Jackie wasn't aware. She'd go ballistic, he knew that. That was probably why he'd eaten when he was out. 'I'm becoming a bloody secret eater now!'

'Mhmm, finding yourself eating in secret.'

Steve shook his head, 'that's not me. I don't like it. But what can I do?'

'It isn't like you to be like that. And you don't like it.'

'I don't. I'm uncomfortable with it. I didn't really enjoy it either time, not really, not deep down, but I just felt the urge and, well, there was nothing to stop me but myself, and I couldn't.'

'That urge took over and you couldn't do anything about it.' John sought to be accepting of what Steve was saying, allowing him to express himself, to not feel pressured by any conditional reaction that might cause him to be less open in his exploration and communication.

'I couldn't. I want to be in control, John. I want to get this right.' He paused. 'Do you think I'm getting a bit too intense about all of this?'

'Can you say a little more, I'm not sure what you mean.'

'Like I'm trying to be too, well, rigid I guess. I mean, I don't want to make a habit of slipping up, but I wish I didn't have to be secretive.'

Steve knows it is the secretive element as well as the fact of knowing how easy it would be to slip back into eating burgers and chips that is worrying him. But he makes an important point about wondering if he is too intense. People can, when seeking to control their eating, become so intense that it actually becomes an eating problem of another kind, the control gets away from them. Somehow a balance needs to be struck, and an acceptance that there may be days when the old pattern, or elements of it, rears up and asserts itself. It can be helpful when a partner understands this from the outset, not so that the client has an excuse, but simply to take the pressure off the client either developing a fanatical intensity and another set of problems, or feeling unable to meet the goals and going into a secretive eating pattern, and in their shame denying this to others.

As an aside, where an over-eating pattern was established early in life in response to some traumatic experience or set of experiences that induced a dissociated state, in extreme cases a person could eat from within such a state, and on emerging from it be unaware that the binge has occurred. Whilst this may be rare, there may be occasions when a person denies eating because the memory is lodged within a dissociated part within their structure of self that they may not normally have awareness of.

'So you'd rather it was out in the open if this happens?'

Steve nodded and then sighed. 'But I guess people slip up. I just can see how easy it would be to make a habit of it.'

'That concern of not making a habit of it seems very present for you.' John was responding to the fact that Steve had mentioned it twice.

'I can see how easy it is – once it's happened. I mean, Friday was maybe a one off, or so it seemed, but on Monday I used Friday to justify it. That was the problem.'

'Like you've got away with it once, so once more won't matter?'

'And that's not good. I have to control that.'

'Mhmm.'

'I want to keep to my changes.'

'You want to keep to your changes.'

'I do, I really do, but I just don't know. It's too easy to eat, too easy to just grab something extra.'

John nodded. 'It's all too easy to just grab something else to eat. What's going to help you, Steve?'

The first part of the response is empathic, but the second part refocuses the client away from the easiness of eating something extra to what he might do about it. That shift would most probably have happened at some point, but in person-centred counselling it is for the client to choose when, and that will be when they have satisfied their exploration of the question of how easy it is to eat something extra. Steve may have had other things to say but he has been directed away from them.

'I don't know. I mean, Jackie knows I'm struggling, but not that I've slipped up a couple of times. I've tried to explain about what happened last week but she finds it hard to understand. It's not that she isn't supportive, she is, she really is. It's me. It's my stuff, my fucking demons that are getting to me. Why do I get so fucking hungry?'

'That questions burns for you, doesn't it?'

'It chews at me. I mean, what we said last week, yes, yes; I can see I ate in the past to feel comfortable, to kind of get that good feeling of being full. I know that, I know it up here.' Steve tapped himself on the side of the head. 'But tell that to my guts, to my stomach down here.'

'Knowing isn't enough, it's like you need to know in your guts as well as your head.'

Steve was feeling more and more frustrated with himself, and angry. 'If this is a direct result of those bastards at school, shit, if I'd known then what I know now, about how what they did would affect me, did affect me, I'd have kicked the fucking shit out of them, all of them.'

'Yeah, if you knew then ...'

Steve was shaking his head. 'I mean, I was pretty angry anyway in those days. Like I've said before, I'd be up for a fight, particularly after a few beers. That's how it was, how I was. Not necessarily proud of it, looking back now, but, well, I can't deny how it was.'

'You needed to do something with that anger, alcohol sort of released it, do you mean?'

'Yeah. Mean, I didn't think of it like that, well, you don't, do you? But yeah, I guess that was how it was.'

'And you can still feel that anger now judging by what you're saying and how you're saying it.'

'And you know, since last week, yeah, I think I've felt more angry. Hadn't quite thought of it like that but, well, yeah, I think that's how it's been. Like I want to lash out, you know?'

'Mhmm, want to lash out at ...'

'I don't know, someone, something, maybe anything. Just want to ...' He paused. 'That's another thing. I seem to want to drink again, I mean, I hadn't stopped as you know, just cut back, but I feel like I want to head down the pub. And, yeah, maybe you're right, maybe that's what it is.'

John wasn't sure quite what Steve thought he had suggested though his assumption was that it was to do with anger and alcohol.

'Right about ... ?'

'Drinking to get angry, or to be angry, maybe ..., maybe ...' Steve thought back over the week. It had been frustrating, he'd had a few problems with a couple of jobs – bloody roofs had leaked on the conservatories they'd fitted. That had pissed him off. The customers had been fairly understanding, he was frustrated with the two who had fitted them. They'd clearly botched it both times. He'd had words. Neither had seemed to want to take it too seriously, he wasn't sure why. Discovered later that they had just been winding him up. But by then he was wound up. Maybe ... he looked over to John. 'Those two bastards I work with, they wound me up. That didn't help. Bastards.'

'So they wound you up and that left you wanting to drink?'

Steve nodded. 'What a bloody week to do it.'

'Not very helpful, of all weeks.' John also had the thought that whilst it hadn't been helpful, so often things like that did happen at the worst time. He'd never really understood why, but he'd heard similar stories of things happening when you least needed them. But maybe it was helping Steve make more sense of his anger and how he coped with it.

> The counsellor has maintained his empathy and the client has moved towards an exploration of his anger, and is more expressive of it in his language. The client feels heard enough to move the focus on to something else.

'So, I've got to keep out of the pub, stop getting angry, and keep myself out of the burger bar.' Steve shook his head. 'Maybe I need something to shrink my stomach. I have wondered about asking my doctor, they do surgery too, don't they? Not sure about that, seen some of those programmes on TV, plastic surgery, euugh, horrid stuff. And all that fat. I saw one a few weeks back, this doctor with a sort of vacuum hose-thing sucking all this yellowy stuff out of a woman's body. They showed it to you in these kinds of bottles. Made me feel sick. She seemed happy to have it done, but, no, not that. I couldn't do that. The way this guy was moving this suction hose around inside her. It was, aaggh, grotesque. No, I'd have to be desperate to have that, and I don't think I'll ever be that desperate.' He paused. 'But I guess some people are, some people really do need that. I feel for them, John, to feel that that is their only option.' He shook his head. 'I suppose I reacted quite strongly to it because, well, that could have been me. What I was seeing coming out of her is what's in me, isn't it?'

> Steve expresses an opinion. Clearly, this is not something that he wants to contemplate for himself. His comments seem derogatory, that is how he feels. However, in reality this form of treatment may be necessary for people with severe morbid obesity and anyone considering this should get professional advice and information as to exactly what is involved along with the clinical benefits of the treatment. Of course, it can only ever remove fat, the person would still need to work on their own processes of psychological and behavioural change in order to maintain the sudden weight loss.

John nodded, maintaining the eye contact with Steve.
'Too much, I don't think I could go for that, but then, I suppose if I was desperate, or had really serious problems and that was the only option.' He shook his head again. 'I don't know. Maybe if that was the only option.'
'Mhmm?'

'No, no, I can't see it. But, well, people who do go for it, good luck to them. I hope it works. I gather, from what they are saying, it helps, but people have to change their eating habits. But, no, too much for me to consider, I think.'

'So that was too much, beyond anything you might consider.'

Steve pulled a face. 'No. But, well, I suppose the thing is, as I say, what they pumped out of her I've got inside me, haven't I?' He pulled a face again. 'Makes me feel sick thinking about it.'

'The thought of all that yellowy fat inside your body makes you feel sick.'

'Oh, geez, don't remind me.'

John felt the temptation to push it, sensing that maybe the feelings Steve had about what he had seen might be a factor that could contribute to his motivation. Should he say something outrageous? He could see Steve's discomfort and revulsion. He didn't need to remind him.

'Being reminded of it makes you feel sick.'

'I tell you, a bottle of that stuff sitting on the table at home, that would stop me eating, I'm bloody sure of it. Particularly if it was mine! I can see the point in that, a sort of reminder to spur you on?'

John had to smile, that was exactly the outrageous thought he'd had. He decided to share it.

'Sorry, Steve, I can't help smiling, but I was just thinking the same thing, and wondering whether to say it.'

'Fuck that. Oh, no, it was 'orrible. No thanks.' He paused, 'But you're probably right, but don't go getting any for me.'

'No, but you need something to make you think twice, a reason to say no when that craving comes on.'

'Well maybe we've found something, maybe I need to remind myself. I should have recorded that programme, you know. But not on a full stomach.'

'So, reminding yourself of that might help?'

Steve looked down at his stomach. 'I like to think there's a lot of muscle down there. I guess I'm kidding myself.'

'Probably.'

There has been some humour in this exchange and in a way the client has needed that because the implication of the television programme for his own body has made an impression. It switches back to seriousness which then takes the client to a further exploration (*see* below) about emptiness.

Also, in the dialogue above, the counsellor allows himself to smile and to be honest about his own thoughts matching those of his client. It's a human moment, the two of them sitting with the same idea. Both know that the idea probably has some merit, the client suggesting, though, that a video recording would have been enough. He now has a graphic image in his mind of what is in his body. It is an image that has meaning to him and will probably not go away. It has strengthened his resolve to find his own way to tackle his weight and his eating.

Steve was still with the image on TV. He appreciated that maybe it might work for some people, but it seemed pretty extreme to him. No, he'd fight it his own way. He sort of felt a little different as well, having just had that conversation. He thought back to the things they'd discussed, and to the previous week's experience. 'I'm still wanting to make sense of that emptiness, I mean, I understand why it was there, and I understand what I did to fill it. I can see all of that. But are you saying that for all of my life I've been carrying round a belly full of emptiness which I keep trying to fill? Is it as simple as that?'

'I'm not sure I'm saying that; seems to be something that you've developed as a way of understanding it, but I'm not going to disagree with the possibility of what you are saying.' That was a bit verbose, John thought, but he didn't want Steve to take on that it was his, John's, explanation. He wanted Steve to make sense of it his way and own whatever conclusion he reached. But he did think that basically Steve had got hold of the essence of it, though it was undoubtedly not that simple.

'I'll take that as a yes, then.' Steve shook his head, though he was smiling.

John smiled back. 'I know that sounded a bit of a mouthful, but I really want you to make sense of it in your own way because that is what will have most meaning for you. You know what it feels like, you know how you've been over the years. I can't know that.'

'Well, I have to say it does make sense. And, yes, I can see that when I started to grow and began to eat more deliberately to build myself up even more, well, yes, that was something else. And it is a habit, no doubt about that. I mean, I don't go around eating because I feel empty, well, not like that. Hungry, yes.'

John was listening closely to what Steve was saying. Yes, it had become a little conversational, yet he felt in contact with Steve, and he had a very clear question take shape in his mind, and it seemed relevant to the dialogue that he and Steve were having. 'Listening to you speak I'm wondering about the difference between eating on feeling hungry, and eating on feeling empty.'

The counsellor has voiced his question, his decision to do so being informed by the fact that his experience of the question is that it has emerged through his therapeutic connection with his client. It is not a personal curiosity. It is important that he is able to recognise if this were to be the case as this would not be reason to voice the question.

Steve thought about it, and he realised that he didn't know. What was the difference? When he was hungry, well, he just knew he wanted something to eat. He wasn't actually, necessarily hungry, he called it being hungry, but he could feel quite full and still be looking for something to snack on. So . . . 'Hmm.'

'Hmm?'

'Well, I was just thinking. I can feel the urge to snack when I'm full, so I can't say I'm feeling hungry although I guess that's what I might say at the time.'

'So, the urge to snack isn't necessarily a hunger urge.'

'No, so maybe that's when there's a kind of emptiness around. I mean, you know, if I'm feeling bored, is that like feeling empty?'

'Is that how you'd describe it, feeling bored being like feeling empty?'

Steve nodded slowly. 'I guess it is. I mean, being bored is like having nothing to do, there's a kind of, well, void I guess. So I fill it, don't I, fill it with food.'

'So you fill the void with food, even though physically you are feeling full. Is that how it is?'

Steve was nodding again. 'Yes, yes that makes perfect sense. I'm sure we've sort of looked at something like this before, we did talk about snacking and boredom, but that was before my experience last week. So, yes, OK, I can see that, feeling empty, not an empty stomach, but a general empty, well, empty life, I suppose? But that sounds harsh. I mean, my life isn't empty. I have lots of things I'm doing, and, no, I wouldn't say it was empty.'

'OK, not empty, but at times not full, would that be reasonable?' John knew that he had lead Steve on, and yet he was experiencing a sense of not full. He did wonder whether he'd got caught up in trying to explain what was happening, and running ahead of the client, not staying with him and letting him describe what he was experiencing. And yet it had felt somehow right to say it. He did feel integrated in the relationship and not centred in his own process and inner experience. He did feel like he was sensing his client's inner world.

This can be OK. Rogers suggested two qualities of empathy, that which is conveying an understanding of what the client is experiencing, and that which conveys a sense of the meaning of what is present within the client's inner world, but which the client has yet to fully grasp for him or herself. He shared the following comment from a client with regard to this: 'Every now and again, with me in a tangle of thought and feeling, screwed up in a web of mutually divergent lines of movement, with impulses from different parts of me, and me feeling the feeling of it being all too much and suchlike – then whomp, just like a sunbeam thrusting its way through cloudbanks and tangles of foliage to spread a circle of light on a tangle of forest paths, came some comment from you. [It was] clarity, even disentanglement, an additional twist to the picture, a putting in place. Then the consequence – the sense of moving on, the relaxation. These were sunbeams' (Rogers, 1957). The counsellor conveys his understanding of his client not feeling his life was empty, but then adds his sense that at times it's not full which may be a meaning that is present but not fully experienced by the client.

Somehow that comment made so much sense. And it left Steve with the idea that he didn't need to be completely empty to experience that urge to eat. It was like, yes, if a part of himself wasn't full, just a part, then maybe that could, would, trigger the urge to eat. So any part of his life that wasn't full, and being bored was one area, but there were many areas of his life. Maybe lots of things that left him not quite full. Somehow, somehow what John had said had shifted his thinking. He needed to think about the parts of his life, the different things that somehow didn't fully satisfy him, that left him somehow, somewhere, to some degree not full. He didn't need to be completely empty. He had felt that way in the past, yes, he could see that. But it wasn't the emptiness that came from being empty, it was the sense of emptiness that came from not feeling full. The hole full of emptiness, that was how it had been. He didn't feel that degree of emptiness these days, well, not until that last counselling session. It all made sense though he knew he had to think it through some more.

John sat, watching Steve as he himself sat with his thoughts. He didn't know what was going on, what his comment had triggered. He waited for Steve to express it, if he chose to do so. He was mindful of wanting to be open to Steve and those words 'shared-into' came back into his mind. He noted them but didn't dwell on them, choosing to maintain his focus and his openness directed towards Steve.

'That really helped, I don't have to be empty, completely empty, the whole of me empty. Yes, that's what I think I felt as a child and that's what came at me last week. I think I have to think about the parts of me, or my life, that don't feel quite full, where something is missing. I think that maybe that's important, that's what I am maybe more sensitive to, those pockets of emptiness, and maybe some are more than pockets, but those are perhaps what make me feel I need to eat. That's where past and present get a bit tangled, but I think I'm making sense. It does to me.'

The session continued a little longer before finally ending, with agreement again for a session the following week. Steve felt more at ease again knowing this, and he was also aware of being quite intrigued as well about what he was thinking about himself.

Points for discussion

- Evaluate the supervision session. Were issues that needed to be addressed brought to the session? What else might you have brought?
- How do you react to the notion of being open to other forms of connection to clients beyond the five senses?
- What were the key therapeutic moments in counselling session 8, and why?
- Identify examples of John's use of congruence.
- Consider Steve and describe his experiencing in terms of person-centred theory, but in your own words.
- How would you relate the content of this session to the processes of change described in Appendices 1 and 2?
- Write notes for counselling session 8.

CHAPTER 5

An update on progress . . .

Following counselling session eight, Steve explored more of this notion of emptiness, realising that it was very much that any part of himself that was not fully satisfied left him sensitive to feeling empty. He commented that it was hard for him to see anything as half-full, or even almost full; rather he was aware of the bit that was missing. It wasn't something he was always aware of, but he noticed it as a kind of theme in his life. What developed from this was Steve making a list – his own idea – of all the experiences that he felt less than satisfied with, that could leave him with that sense of not being full, and started to consider how these were related to urges to eat. It wasn't easy to differentiate; he was still experiencing a general overall urge to eat that was still very much the legacy from the session when he had so powerfully connected with those feelings of emptiness and sadness. Nevertheless, he persevered, and over the next few weeks, gained a great deal of insight into himself.

He continued to lose weight and was now down to eighteen stone. It is now three months later and Steve has returned back to fortnightly counselling sessions. It is counselling session 16 and he had suggested at the end of the last session that it would be good to just review things in the following session. John had agreed to this. Steve had been thinking, when he had suggested this, about not only revisiting his eating triggers, but also to consider his future goals and aims.

Counselling session 16: a review, looking forward and acknowledging responsibility

'So, you said last time that you wanted to review things this week, take stock of the situation and think about future goals.'

'I've been taking time to reflect on what has been happening. There's the weight, of course, and I'm glad it's coming down. And I do want to lose more, and I think I feel more OK about that, now. I don't think that mentally and emotion-ally I need to carry the weight around the same as I know that I did before.' Steve was thinking about how his size had been such an important part of who he was, but that was changing. It had helped that he and Jackie were now extending their social lives more.

'So your sense of who Steve is has changed.'

Steve nodded. 'And it's a weird one in many ways, not easy to really describe but I know there's a change. And I do feel better in myself. The mood swings that I went through have eased and I feel more stable, calmer in myself. Those ses-sions where I got angry, I really think they helped me to let go of that. It's not that I don't still get angry, I do, but there's a greater acceptance as well.'

'Acceptance?'

'Of myself, I guess.'

'So, you feel more accepting of you, you as you are now?'

'Yes, but maybe not just that.' Steve was frowning. He was thinking back to his past. 'I mean, I don't think I found it always easy to accept me as the person I was. I hated being bullied, being weak and vulnerable and I vowed never to be like that once I got bigger and stronger. And that was something I have carried with me until recently, when, with your help, I've realised that I don't need to be like that any more. But that's been a hard one to let go of. And I'm not sure that I fully have. I still don't want to feel vulnerable. I know what it's like, and I don't want that again.'

'Yes, that's very clear, you know what it is like to be vulnerable and, as you say, you don't want that experience again.'

'But what I have realised is that my size isn't the only way of not feeling vulner-able. It's also about stuff in my head as well.'

'About the way you think?'

'I'm still big, and I will probably always be big, but not as big. It was the extreme that was unnecessary, although at the time it was who I was and how I felt I needed to be.' He paused, thinking about what he had said. 'Well, I suppose that's not strictly true. I wasn't thinking about it like that, rather it was how it was, how I'd become. And I can sort of understand now why I became the way that I did, but it's still hard to accept how I was, particularly when I was caught up in all the violence through the football. I really was a mean bastard in those days, and I can see that I had so much anger in me, bottled up from those early years. And then, as we discussed, it did become a habit, in fact more like an addiction – the buzz, the thrill, the adrenalin, being part of a group of people and being respected for what I was – well, what I had become. Now, well, now I wouldn't want that kind of respect.'

'That respect was important then, but not now.'

The counsellor is empathising with the concluding remark, not trying to empathise with all that has been said, allowing the client to stay with his flow and process of thinking and feeling.

'It was very important.' Another pause. 'I mean, I'd go so far as to say that I lived for it. They were crazy times. We were a bunch of nutters, I can see that. And thank God I came out of it, and I really have to thank Jackie for that. She really did make an impact on me.' He shook his head and felt a surge of emotion. He really loved her, and the counselling had made him more aware of, more sensitive to, that love. 'We have difficult times, of course we do, who doesn't? But we're good for each other, and we really do encourage each other. We both want more healthy lives, and a future together. It's really important to us. That's another big change, looking ahead.'

'Looking ahead?'

'I didn't think ahead much as a young man, and I'm not sure that Jackie and I did, not so much as we do now. I know I didn't. It was live for the day and you just assumed tomorrow would be the same, and that was OK.' He shook his head, tightening his lips as he did so. 'Now, well, now that's not good enough. We are thinking ahead. And maybe my health problems helped, although at first I'm not sure how much I wanted to think ahead because it seemed like I had to accept that I didn't know what the future would be. I didn't really talk about that, but it was scary. Those breathless episodes have stopped now, unless I really overdo it. But, well, I can understand that. But I am getting fitter, and I'd say stronger – you don't need weight to be strong, do you?'

John shook his head.

'So I am looking forward to the future now. We're also thinking of joining a language class in the autumn. That will be a new thing for both of us. We've decided to go for Spanish, and feel that it will be something we can do together, and that it'll not only be an evening out, it will also be something we'll share in the home as well. We're both looking forward to it but neither of us feels particularly confident. But it means that we can maybe use the language for holidays.'

'That sounds very exciting, and I can hear that uncertainty over how it will be.'

'I didn't pay much attention to languages at school, Jackie did a bit of French, but found it difficult, so we really are starting out. Even if it's too much, we'll learn something and, well, I hope it won't be like school too much.'

John knew from his own experience that evening language classes could be fun, and were generally much more relaxed and more creative than his memory of language classes at school. 'I think you'll find it different.'

'You've done any, then?'

'I went for Italian for a few years. It was good. Our teacher was Italian, I found that really helpful. She really brought a flavour of Italy into the lessons. It was fun.' John felt the self-disclosure was acceptable. The relationship had moved on quite a lot and there were now times when it was more conversational.

When does a person-centred counsellor offer a self-disclosure? When it is either emerging out of the therapeutic relationship or, as in this case, conveys information that the client may find helpful. The latter, however, needs care. It has to be owned and is not telling the client what they can expect.

In this instance it is also conveyed in a manner that is suggestive that the therapeutic relationship is well established and there can be times when the dialogue enters into more conversational phases. That is fine, there are times when the client will need that. However, it should not be allowed to dominate otherwise the counsellor moves away from offering empathy and something else replaces it. Having said that, an empathic understanding of a client's need might lead to the recognition that a client actually needs to experience conversation rather than therapy, and perhaps the therapeutic relationship may be the place they find it most easy to develop conversational skills.

'That's good to hear.' Steve paused before returning to his previous theme. 'So, we are looking ahead, thinking more about what we want longer term. One thing is that we have been considering having a family. May seem strange after all this time, but I've been the one who has been reluctant. I know we talked about this before as it is an area that I know is part of my sense of emptiness. And I didn't want a family because I wasn't at all sure that I'd be any good as a father, and I was really concerned about . . . , well, the kind of experiences I had.'

John nodded. He appreciated what Steve was trying to say. 'You wouldn't want a child of yours to go through it.'

Steve shook his head. 'And I've come to realise that, well, that's really selfish. Jackie wants to be a mother, of course she does. And although she is a little bit younger than me, we don't want to leave it too late. And that's a really big step. But it's been difficult, as you know.'

'It sounds as though together you have made a big decision and for you, Steve, you've realised that you want children.'

'It's about my identity again, as well, about wanting to be a father. I do. It scares me as well, but I do.'

John nodded. 'It's a scary idea but it's what you want, what you both want.'

'It'll be good for us too, but that's not the reason.'

'Mhmm. You're not doing it for the sake of your marriage?'

'No. No, we're good together anyway, but it'll add something more.' Steve smiled, suddenly feeling a little more uncertain. It showed in his facial expression.

'Still a bit uncertain, or maybe that's not the right word for the expression I can see on your face.'

'It's something new. I don't know how I'll be.'

'The newness and not knowing how you will be, that's what makes it feel the way that it does?'

Steve nodded. 'So, there's that. And the other thing that I really wanted to just I suppose talk about is the way that, as we discussed in earlier sessions, how I eat on emptiness, how my sense of not being satisfied with something, anything, leaves me with an urge to eat. That's much more under control. It's been really helpful these past few weeks keeping a close eye on that. It really has amazed me just how many things make me feel like eating. Something doesn't go well at work – eat something. Frustrated by traffic delays – eat something. Plan a day out and it rains – eat something. Just feel tired when you want to feel alert – eat something. It goes on and on. It's like eating became my answer to everything, at least, not so much an answer to the thing, whatever it was, but to how I felt. Worrying about something? Eat. And it was always junk food in the past, or the sweet stuff. Now, well, now the urge is still there, but we have healthier things in the house. I used to go for crisps, now we have nuts, or nuts and raisins, or tropical mixes, things like that, but they're not out all the time. So it's not that I'm eating vast amounts, but I really need to try and quell that urge. The trouble is, the temptation is then to have more, and I've realised the best thing is to try and have nothing, or actually fruit. That helps as well.'

'So, you have some healthier options, but the urge can still be there, and it can get out of control.'

Steve nodded. 'It's like, when that urge really fires up, it really is powerful. And I tell myself that it can't be hunger, not real hunger. I eat enough to not need to feel hungry, so I know it's this other stuff setting me off.'

'So, the urge to eat you can see isn't real hunger in the sense of not having had enough food.'

'No, I know it's what I learned in the past, and I know to some degree it's still there. But as I get more variety into my life, and as Jackie and I do more together, well, we encourage each other not to eat something. It's been really helpful that a lot of this has been happening at this time of year. We do go for walks a lot now. Something I'd never have thought of doing – something old people do! Well, that's what I thought, but actually it isn't like that at all. And getting Sam [the dog] was something else that just made a difference, gave us a focus, something to think about and a reason to go for walks. That's made a huge difference, mind you, he eats like crazy and we're having to keep an eye on him. But he gets plenty of exercise.'

John was sitting with a lot of thoughts and feelings in response to the way Steve was talking. He felt he wanted to share them.

It is appropriate for a counsellor to share their thoughts and feelings when there is a sense of it having therapeutic value. John has been listening to Steve tell him about the positive changes that have happened in his life, and it almost demands a human response and acknowledgement from him. At the same time, Steve might also say more about how it is all leaving him feeling.

'Hearing you speak just leaves me with a lot of thoughts and feelings, and I guess you think and feel differently because of all that is happening. I just want to say that it makes me feel really great hearing you talk like this. And that's not to in any way sound negative about how you spoke in the past, at the beginning.

You spoke then as you needed to speak. It was the start of the process. Now, well, now things have moved on, you have moved on, and it is great to see.'

Steve felt slightly embarrassed yet he also knew that John was right and it was good to hear how he felt. It was a kind of affirmation. Yes, he did feel different and it sort of validated it a bit more knowing that John saw that difference too. 'Thanks for that. I really think you've been a life saver, and I do mean that sincerely.'

John felt emotional hearing Steve say that. He hadn't quite thought of it that way. And he knew it wasn't down to him. His role was in enabling Steve to be more aware of himself, to become more whole, less the victim of his introjects and the 'conditions of worth' that developed earlier in his life, and later to some degree as well.

'I feel humbled. Thanks, I'm glad to have contributed, and I want to say that you're the one who, twenty-four/seven is having to make fresh choices, to make and sustain the changes that you have embarked on.'

Steve sat for a moment, wondering where he might have been had he not been detailed off to counselling by his GP. 'I was so reluctant to come at the start, I really thought that maybe I'd have that one session, tell the doctor I'd done what he said, but it didn't work. I really didn't want to change, although somewhere in me I must have known that I had to. It just seemed too much to want to think about. The idea of change was too much. The consequences of not changing were too much.'

'And that can be the problem, everything is too much and you sort of do nothing, or it gets worse because you now have more to be worried about.'

'You remember how my eating went up?'

'Mhmm, and you got angry with me because of it.'

'Yes, well, I had to blame someone.'

'Yes, and you did.'

'But it was me, me that I needed to blame, but didn't want to blame. I couldn't take responsibility. I couldn't.'

'No.'

'It was someone or something else's fault. And in a way it was. I held on to what I felt about myself. And I can see that, yes, I was a victim, and I did what I needed to do to get some kind of satisfaction from my life, some kind of relief from the horrible feelings that were around. I comfort ate. I became a bully. They were my choices though I didn't really have any control. And I could carry on, eating and bullying to feel better. I did. But I never stopped to think. I never stopped to feel, either. And when I did, fuck me, that session where I really lost it, you remember, when I really experienced that sadness and loneliness for the first time.'

'Mhmm, I remember.'

'That was, well, that was a turning point. And somehow I gradually realised that I had to take responsibility. That I could make different choices, not just because the doctor said I should, or because I didn't want the consequences if I didn't, but because I wanted something different. My choices, down to me. And being a different me to make those choices.'

John was nodding. He really appreciated what Steve was saying and how he was saying it. 'You really express all this very clearly, you really have taken on board your need to change and to act differently.'

'And to think and feel differently. It's everything isn't it?'

'Mhmm.'

'I mean, I thought I was coming to just talk about my weight, but, well, it's everything. My weight was like a symptom of other things.'

'Pretty much, as well as being a health problem itself.'

'It's been really good having this session. I really felt I needed this time to just talk about it all like this, take stock of where I've been and what I've achieved. And now, well, now it's about looking ahead.'

'Mhmm. Rewiew the past, the changes, take stock of your achievements and then, turn to face forwards.'

'That's very much it, turning to look ahead. My life has been dominated by my past without me really being aware of it. Everything driven by what happened then, and so easy to just keep it going, or at least, keep the effects going.'

John nodded. 'They had become your reality, and we don't change our reality often unless we are pushed to do so.'

'I was pushed, and then I had to push myself, and you, well, I'm not sure whether you pushed or not. I certainly felt a push, but it wasn't like you were telling me what to do, you weren't like a doctor.'

'So, you felt pushed but not a sense that I was pushing, is that what you mean?'

'Yes, I was pushing myself. But you were a big part in that.' Steve paused. Yes, he thought, you've been doing something here to make me change, but most of the time you've just listened, occasionally throwing in a suggestion, but generally just listening, helping me make sense of myself and why I behave the way that I do.

John let the comment go and waited for Steve to continue.

'So, the question of what next.'

'Yes. What do you want to look at?'

'I want to lose a bit more weight, but probably aim now for sixteen stone as a final weight. I know that's still some way off, but I feel that's what I want to work towards. It feels reachable and somehow appeals. I don't know why. It has a substantial feel to it and, well, that's important.' Steve wasn't totally sure why, but it just felt like a good weight, at least for now. 'Maybe I might change my mind when I get there! But I need to perhaps contain what I eat a little more, though I do think I have a much more normal diet. Actually, it's healthier than what many people would call normal. I know that.'

'So it feels quite healthy but you sense you could eat a little less?'

'I think that, apart from snacks, and they really are pretty much out of the picture, apart from the odd handful of nuts, or fruit, it's about portions. It really is. There's always been a sense of wanting to have a full plate and that's been a tough one. We reduced the size of the plates, but that didn't feel right, didn't feel like a proper plate somehow. I know it's all crazy stuff in my head, but size matters!' Steve smirked as he spoke.

John could not, and did not try, to contain his own smile. 'Not sure what to say to that. So I'll just agree with you.'

Steve was still smiling. 'It's bloody true, though.'

'So the size of the plate and the size of the portion.'

'And I have cut back, and, well, there's just still something good about a big plateful, I don't care what people say, that's how it is.'

'Mhmm, a big plateful is a satisfying experience?'

'Yes, and if it isn't a big plateful then that stuff about feeling empty cuts in. It still happens. I can control it more, but it happens.'

'Before or after you've eaten?'

'Both, but very much before.'

'So, you look at that plateful, it's not big enough, and then in comes that feeling of emptiness.'

'It's not so much that I feel empty, it's hard to describe, but it's associated with that, it's like a sort of "ohh" from somewhere inside me.'

'Ohh'. John dropped his voice and tone as he repeated back what Steve had said, matching his way of pronouncing it.

'It's sort of disappointing, you know? A bit like – and I can remember this, and it still happens sometimes, you're in a restaurant and you make a choice. It's a difficult choice, two meals, each sounding really good. You think you've made a good one. Then you see the meal you didn't choose being served to someone else. It looks good, but you know yours will be better, at least, that's what you hope. What you are secretly also feeling is that yours will be bigger. And it comes. And it isn't, and there's that "ohh" moment of disappointment. You want to change the order. It's suddenly not fair. You don't want to admit to having made the wrong choice, that would be to accept responsibility. It's the restaurant's fault, they should have told you, there should be a symbol on the menu – they tell you what is vegetarian, they should rank the meals in order of size. You've been conned. But it's their fault, they've made it happen and you've become their victim.'

'I notice that more with desserts, but I do know what you mean.'

'Yes, desserts too. Yes, you order something and it sounds big, ice-cream, fruit, cream, biscuits. You know you've made the right choice. Out it comes and there it is, on a big plate. Two very small scoops of ice-cream, a few berries placed artistically on the plate, a zig-zag of something red, and a small blob of that disgusting cream they squirt out of a can, frothed whitewash I call it. And the person next to you gets a bucket of ice-cream, with chocolate pieces, cream, nuts, wafers, the works. And they know they've got what you want, you can see it in their face as they look at yours and say, with a smirk, "yours looks very nicely laid out". Bastard. You know?'

John nodded. He knew exactly what Steve meant. Steve, he could conjure up such a wonderful image when it came to food. 'Yeah, I know.'

Steve was on a roll. 'And they keep looking at you as they take another mouthful, and you're picking at yours, desperate to make it last. You don't want to be sitting there with an empty plate whilst they are still digging down, like some crazed archaeologist, into the depths of their bucket, gently excavating it, eyeing each mouthful with glee before putting it in their mouths. And you know, if you finish first, they'll say, between mouthfuls, "that did look nice. Did it taste good? Were you pleased with your choice?" And you just want to bury their head in their dessert.'

'Sounds like you've had a lot of experience.'

'Oh yes, and I've had the large ice-cream sundae, and I've savoured it and watched some other poor bastard push his biscuit round the plate.' Steve was still grinning as he spoke.

'Good feeling, huh?'

'Wonnn-derful.'

'You know, it feels good hearing you joke about food like this. I mean, I know it's serious, but there is a time for lightness as well.'

'I know. There's just so much that happens around a table like that, so many unvoiced feelings. I love it, so long as I get the decent portions, of course!'

'Of course. Well, on that note we need to end, Steve. Time is almost up. Has this review and reminiscence been helpful?' John couldn't resist throwing in the reminiscence.

'Yes, it has. And there's no problem in carry on coming?'

'No, you still have a goal to work towards, and that's fine by me.'

'OK, couple of weeks again, and then there'll be a gap because I have two weeks holiday, starting the week that I'd have seen you after the next one.'

'OK, so I see you in two weeks then you are away for two weeks, so the next one would be after three weeks.'

'And I think next time it would be good to talk about being on holiday. It's the first long break away since I started all this, and, well, holidays have been an excuse to eat and drink in the past. Though I am trying to avoid that, but . . .'

'Sure, we'll look at that next time.'

Supervision: exploring what person-centred means inside and out of counselling

'Steve's still doing really well, Chloe. He's sticking at it, and he seems to be contemplating more serious changes in his life.'

'Such as?'

'Starting a family.'

'So, looking ahead more, do you think?'

'That came up. Yes, he's aware of that, of being able to think of the future rather than be simply affected by his past.'

'And for you, how does that feel?'

'Good. Encouraging. It's heartening to hear. I said something about how it left me feeling when he talked about changes and looking ahead.'

'And how did he receive it?'

'I thought well.Yes, yes, I felt he took it on board. Not that I want him to evaluate his success on what I say, I want him to feel it and own it for himself, which I think he does.'

'So, all in all, it's very satisfying.'

'Yes, and he made reference again to that feeling empty, and we had a bit of a review session really, it was a bit lighter, which was good. He talked about the different experiences that can leave him with an urge to eat, things going wrong, not working out as he had planned, things that are generally unsatisfying to him in some way.'

'And he still experiences that?'

'Yes, to some degree, but he's more aware of it, more able to make different choices. And he said about having healthier options if he does want to eat something nuts, fruit, that kind of thing. But he also talked about how there was a difference between feeling hungry because he hadn't eaten enough, and the urge to eat because he was unsatisfied. He's really differentiating his eating urges. And he wants to continue and bring his weight down more, sixteen stone is his target now. And, well, I think he'll do it, but he has a holiday coming up and he wants to talk about that in the next session. He's saying that it might be difficult – holidays were a time for a lot of eating and drinking by the sound of it.'

'So, first holiday with his new eating and drinking regime.'

'Yes. I don't know any more, he didn't say where or what they were doing. But he's unsure enough to mention it, so I can see what his concerns are and maybe he can formulate some ideas to minimise the risk of a lapse.'

'Tough time when you are on holiday. All your normal routines go. And if you are in a hotel it's so tempting to eat, and often you get substantial meals.'

'Yes, I don't know what they're doing, I'll no doubt hear next time.'

'So, you say you had a review with him, how do you want to use time now?'

'Maybe the same would be helpful. I'd like to talk about how I feel working with him and then maybe explore a little around "eating configurations", as I think that's a new area and one that intrigues me.'

'OK, where do you want to start?'

'Me, how it is to be with Steve. He makes me laugh. He really is quite a raconteur when he gets going.'

'Mhmm, how does that affect you?'

'It feels good, but it does take me away from a therapeutic focus.'

'So, you don't feel you are as therapeutic?'

'I'm not sure. I think what is happening is therapeutic, but I wonder if I relax and maybe I may miss something.'

'How do you mean?'

'I can feel entertained, I'm more an audience, and that isn't what I'm there for.'

'So, more like being a member of an audience when he's, let's say, "entertaining".'

'And it's good to hear him speak like that, he feels good, and maybe some would declare it as being a defence to be challenged, but I don't think so, not at this stage in the counselling process. It feels right for it to lighten up, loosen up, and that isn't to say it won't get heavy and serious again, I'm sure that it will. I suppose I just want to explore my reaction and whether I might, in some way, encourage him to be ..., well, I was going to say to be something other than a client.'

'He has to be a particular way to be a client?' Chloe had a quizzical look on her face, and had raised her eyebrows.

'No, it is for him to be as he wants or needs to be. No, but it can push me into another place.'

'So, let's be specific here, the entertainer in him brings out the audience member in you?'

John thought about it and nodded. 'Yes, and when I'm in that then I'm not sure how much I'm being a therapist.'

'OK, let's take this a stage further. What are you there to be?'

'A therapist.'

'Just a therapist?'

'No, I'm there to be me, a person.'

'OK, so you are there as a person, more than a therapist?'

'I am there as a person in the role of a therapist, and applying a particular approach.'

'OK, so your primary identity is as a person, as John, but it is a John applying the discipline of being a person-centred therapist. Yes?'

'Yes.' He paused. 'Yes, I am being me but within a context. I am being a set of values and seeking to convey certain attitudes and qualities.'

'Which you are as a person or as a therapist or both?'

'Both. Very definitely. I don't see the person-centred approach as being something you switch into. I may switch into being a therapist, but the values of the person-centred approach I take with me into my life outside of the therapy room as well.'

'So, you don't switch person-centred on and off, you carry it with you.'

'I hope it's more than carry it with me, I hope that I am, well, yes, a person-centred person.'

'Mhmm. So you bring your person-centred way of being into the discipline of the therapeutic hour, so to speak, or the therapeutic relationship.'

'That's what I try to do. I try generally in life to be empathic, to be authentic, and to feel warmth for people without it being conditional. I may not always achieve that, but I certainly aim for that. And then in therapy, in counselling, when I'm in counsellor role, then I would say that I am more attentive to those core attitudes, it's not so much a switching on as a tuning up.'

'OK, that's clear, like you carry it anyway, but you tune it up when you are the counsellor?'

John sat thinking for a few moments. Yes, he was quite happy with that, he did bring his person-centredness into the therapeutic relationship, but it was more focused, yes, and more focused on the client. He needed to add that qualification. 'Yes, and I sort of shift my focus. As the person-centred me out in the world I will be more centred on me, on my personness – if there is such a word which I don't think there is – my personhood, that's what I mean.'

'More focused on you, on your experience of being you, do you mean?'

'Yes. I'm living my life for me, for what satisfies me. Not in a selfish way, of course, just in trying to be close to who I am and to live authentically with my own process and experiencing.'

'Sure. Seeking to be authentically yourself and open to what you experience.'

'But as a therapist my focus is on the client – hence client-centred although, I have to say, I still prefer to think of my client as a person than a client.'

'OK, so your focus is then on the client but with a context or attitude of thinking about the client as a person.'

'I know they are in a client role as I am in a counsellor role, but I also want to minimise that. We are two people, two persons, but we are not two people as we would be if we were, say, friends sitting in a café, or strangers chatting on a bus.'

'So the context obviously affects how, as a person, you are and how you perceive the person you are with.'

'And as a person-centred counsellor I bring a certain set of expectations of how I will be. How the client will be, I do not know, but I would be foolish to deny that I carry assumptions and expectations based on past experience, however much I remind myself that my client is a unique individual.'

'So, you have your expectations of you and accept that, however much you might try to minimise it, you will also have some expectations of your client, however minimal.'

'I think so. So for me what is important is that I can be clear that my person-centredness when I am being a counsellor is just that; that the counselling role does not in some way inhibit it, which it does because I know that the person I am in the café with a friend won't be made available to me in the same way when I am counselling. Yes, that's what it is. Does being a person-centred counsellor inhibit my experience of myself as a person-centred person, and I believe it does, and is that OK, and how far should that go?'

'How inhibiting to your personhood is the discipline of being a person-centred counsellor.'

'Yes.' John was quite matter of fact in the way that he spoke. 'That, for me, has become something that not so much intrigues me as demands my attention.'

'And something about your experience with Steve flagged this up?'

'Being in an audience. I'd be like that with a friend, with a stranger in conversation, but as a counsellor? I'm not going to deny the experience, it is there, it is how I can be, it is part of my personhood, but by allowing that to be visibly present, is that OK, or am I doing my client a disservice?'

'And you think you are?'

'I don't know. When it happened with Steve, I didn't think so, but . . . , maybe. I let myself be entertained, but I could have empathised, stayed in counsellor role, but I didn't.'

'I don't want this to sound like a cop out, it's not meant to be, but is this a case for considering situational empathy?'

'How do you mean?'

'Empathy to the situation or context. What did Steve need from you during that exchange of dialogue?'

'He wanted an audience.'

'And that's what you gave him. You honoured his need by your response.'

'OK, maybe, but I wasn't doing it as a therapist, I wasn't thinking – I will honour Steve's need for an audience and therefore show empathy for his need.'

'OK, so maybe that's the key, then. Your response might have been a therapeutic decision, but in that instance your experience was that it wasn't, and that's what is with you?' Chloe was deliberately questioning in her tone, feeling she had grasped what John's issue was, but not totally sure she had captured it accurately.

'Yes, yes, that's it. That's exactly it. Yes. It's OK to be an audience to my client, but only if I am coming from my counselling discipline in that decision, not from my undisciplined self that just naturally flows into that place. Yes. Outwardly, I might behave the same, but inwardly, the motivation is different and the place is different, and I would imagine the quality and nature of my attention, receptivity and communication will be different.'

'Interesting issue, John. So the need to be aware of whether your responses to a client are coming from within your disciplined counselling personhood, or you as you would be at any other time.'

'It's the kind of thing I need to think more about and self-monitor in sessions, and directly after, to try and get a sense of what happens for me.'

'It feels like it could open up a wealth of self-awareness and self-understanding.'

'OK, that's good. Thanks for that. I feel like I want to take that away and ponder and, as I say, be more attentive to myself as a result. And then come back and maybe explore it further.'

'Sure.'

John paused. Chloe was aware that John had mentioned eating configurations earlier, and wondered if he was still wanting to consider that. John, meanwhile, was thinking of another client.

'I'd like to move on to another client.'

'OK, but can I just check – you did say about "eating configurations", or do you want to leave that for another time?'

'Leave that for another time. I do need to spend time on a couple of other clients today. That isn't so pressing.'

The topic of discussion and exploration moved on to John's other clients.

Points for discussion

- Evaluate the therapeutic effectiveness of John's responses in counselling session 16.
- What role does a more conversational tone have in therapeutic counselling? When is it appropriate, and when not?
- What is the therapeutic role of humour?

- What have you taken from the supervision session? If you were John, how might it have helped you in your work with Steve?
- What are your thoughts and feelings about being person-centred in life generally, and being a person- or client-centred counsellor? How do they overlap for you? Can you define your boundaries? Do you have boundaries?
- How would you relate the content of this session to the processes of change described in Appendices 1 and 2?
- Write notes for counselling session 16.

CHAPTER 6

Counselling session 17: holiday preparation and an 'eating dream' explored

John was mindful from the start of the next session with Steve as to the issue that had been discussed in supervision. He felt more strongly, having reflected on it further, that he needed to be clear that his responses and behaviour were responses from within his presence as a self-disciplined, person-centred counsellor.

Steve had begun the session describing the last two weeks, that a few more pounds had come off, that he was trying to reduce his portions further, and had taken the decision to really make sure his alcohol intake was the minimum. A couple of pints now and then was what he wanted to establish. It had been that four or five times a week. That was still a big change from the past, but it had crept up a bit recently and he wanted to bring it back down.

'Ideally, I'd like to just have the odd pint, maybe with a meal, but to stop going out to drink. That's the killer. Going out, a whole evening, and the idea is to fill it with drinking. That's no good to me, not any more.'

'So, a need for a totally different style of drinking.'

'More mature, so to speak,' Steve smiled.

John felt the pull to go into audience mode but he stepped away from it. 'Sort of makes you smile the thought of a mature drinking style?'

'It does, never thought in the past I'd ever say anything like that. But I've settled down. Those days are gone. It is about being more mature and, like I said last time, about responsibility – for my choices and my future.'

'More of a sense of responsibility.'

'That's why I need to talk about this holiday. Two weeks in Madeira. Nice hotel, probably hire a car, not sure whether we need to, but we probably will, and planning to try and keep control of what I eat.'

John nodded. He'd been to Madeira. What should he do, disclose it? He knew a few tips, but at the same time, was that appropriate? He decided to let it ride for the moment, and keep the focus on what Steve was saying.

'So, it's about how to keep control?'

'We've decided to have bed and breakfast and maybe book evening meals when we are there, not sure what we will want to do. It's near the beach, and we want to have some relaxing time, but I need to make sure we keep walking too. The brochure said it's really good for walks, talks about things called levadas, I think that's the word, irrigation streams that you can walk by, and they're fairly flat which is good. But I think we'll need a car to get to them.'

John decided to disclose that he had been there, feeling that it might help Steve to plan his trip and perhaps have ideas around controlling his eating. He was sure it wasn't coming from a need to tell him he'd been there, it felt much more that his motivation was practical and in the hope that it would be helpful.

'You will need a car. I've been there.'

'Oh, right, so what are these levadas like?'

'Really good, long gentle walks around the mountains. Take a torch, there are unlit tunnels through the hillsides.' John also thought of how some of them were quite low and John would have to bend over a little. Oh well, he wasn't going to say anything to discourage him. Not all the walks had tunnels.

'Oh, that sounds intriguing. And food?'

'Lots of fish. Plenty of places to eat. I guess it's about planning your day.'

'So there's a lot to see?'

'Yes, yes there is. A place to take your time as you go round.'

'I suppose so long as we keep to two meals and have something light at lunchtime, that'll be for the best.'

'Mhmm.'

'We'll need to maybe get ourselves into the countryside, if we go for walks and just take water, then we can't be tempted, can we?'

'No, that sounds like a good idea.'

'And there's plenty to see?'

'Oh yes, lots of little towns or villages, mountains, waterfalls.'

'We're staying in Funchal.'

'That's on the sunny side. Botanic Gardens are worth a visit. Watch out for the tea shops, though!'

'Yes, they won't be easy. We've decided to limit ourselves. Not to say no completely, but to have a limit for the holiday. That felt more realistic.'

'Mhmm, yes.'

'And there's Madeira cake and wine, of course.'

'You'll have to sample it, part of being there.'

'Yes, but maybe we need to make that a treat to look forward to rather than get into the habit of it too soon. I don't know. And I don't want to think about it so much that it ruins the holiday.'

'Yes, too much worry about what not to eat and drink and that takes over.'

'That's not the point at all. No, we want to really enjoy the place and make that the focus. Walking, sitting on the beach, sight-seeing, touring. Ice-creams will be another issue. Oh well, holidays.'

'Mhmm. What would be a successful outcome, Steve? What would make you feel, yes, good holiday and now get on with the lifestyle changes?'

'Well, realistically, I'm not going to lose weight those two weeks, but if I can stabilise that would be an achievement. We have to keep getting exercise, and
really not get into habits of stopping for teas, coffees, and the temptations of
cakes and things.'

'So, have alternatives with you and, like you said before, try and give yourself
a limit.'

'I think a limit is more realistic than saying no. Of course we're going to see places
that will look nice and we'll want to stop at. And, well, as I say I know that to
not stop, for me at any rate, will be unsatisfying and I'll get that empty urge to
eat, I can just see it happening. So I've got to be sensible and I guess negotiate
my way through it.'

'So, it's about trying to ensure that you choose things that give you satisfaction?
Lots of fresh fruit there; oranges, banana trees.'

'Well, yes, take bagfuls with us, that kind of thing, anything that means I keep
control but it doesn't spoil the experience.'

'Sure.'

'So, yes, if I haven't put on any weight when we get back, well, I think it'll actually be one hell of an achievement. Realistically, maybe I'll put on half a stone,
maybe. I hope not, but, well, I know what holidays are like.'

'Well, if you do, you know what you'll need to do when you get back to take it
off again.'

'That's it, isn't it, and I guess the risk is that any holiday in future it'll go back up
and I have to bring it back down.'

'That's what it seems like, yeah, is that what you expect?'

'Yes, but no, it does come down again and again to the amount I eat. I just have to
stick to less. That's the reality. It's not as though I'm going to starve myself. I
eat carefully these days, and it is generally healthier food. We're not eating processed foods very much. No, it's still quantity, that's what I have to break the
habit with. Exercise and avoiding the sweet and fattening snacks is working,
but it's still about the amount on my plate. I've changed what I put on it, and
have to some degree changed how much, but I have to change more.'

'That sounds pretty clear, still a matter of amount.'

'It's funny really, can make me hungry talking about food. I leave here sometimes
craving something, but not always. But then, we don't always talk about food.'

'It can be a problem, the way we talk about food?'

'Take last week, after what I was saying, I just craved a bloody ice-cream. Could I
get it out of my head? It was a hot day, remember, that didn't help. But I managed not to have one. Had cold water, wasn't the same, but it filled me up. The
craving can be so, so, oh what's the word?'

'That craving it's just there, so . . .'

'Sharp, but that's not the word. It's like it's, yes, so precise, you know? It's almost
surgical. You know what you suddenly want and it's with you.'

'Like the ice-cream?'

'Yes, but sometimes for something else. Yes, that's a point, it can seem really specific, and, yes, maybe that's different. I used to just be hungry for anything,

yes, now it is more precise. Maybe a bit more refined? Who am I kidding! No, I can get the urge for a bacon butty, like anyone else, I guess, but it's like whatever it is just becomes so present, and so persistent. It really is more precise these days.'

'More precise, more sort of selective?'

'Yes, and it is more intense. I mean, it was intense before, but a more general intense, a sort of more general urge to eat, still a craving, but not so, as you say, selective or specific.'

'So you have become more hungry for a particular something rather than just being hungry for, well, anything?'

'That's right. Chocolate will suddenly be there. I hardly eat chocolate now, and then suddenly I'm thinking about it. Or, what else, maybe a pie of some kind. I'll get a taste for something, maybe apple, or blackcurrant, and it does take a while to pass. It will pass, but it takes time.'

'Do you dream of eating?' John was wondering whether Steve experienced 'eating dreams'. He wasn't quite sure why he had asked the question, it just came to him.

There are times when a counsellor is moved to say something, without knowing quite why, but it sort of feels right. It is a question of professional judgement as to whether it is appropriate, and a major part of that will be how connected the counsellor felt to the client when the urge to speak arose.

People do experience dreams associated with habits that they are trying to change. The notion of 'drinking dreams', for instance (Bryant-Jefferies, 2001). People can re-live drinking experiences in their sleep, waking up with sensations that were associated with alcohol use even though they know they have been abstinent for some while. It can be very disorientating and unsettling and can trigger relapses.

'Funny you should say that, yes, and it was weird. It was incredibly real and I felt like I had eaten. I was out somewhere and had this great big plate full of a mixed grill, all kinds of things, you know, anything and everything that you would include. And I remember eating it and having this battle with myself whilst I was doing so. Yes, I'm really glad you mentioned it, it had got lost somewhere. And I remember feeling it was wrong, thinking that I don't do this, but I was. And I woke up, and I felt full. That was strange. I felt as though I had actually eaten, even though I hadn't. And it sort of left me feeling hungry, or at least, left me thinking about food. I really wasn't sure what had happened when I woke up. Like it took me a while to come to my senses?'

'Mhmm, that sounds like the kind of dream people can have. It can leave people with the taste of food that they haven't eaten for the longest while, and vividly so.'

'I can really believe that. So, yes, yes, that was quite a dream. I don't think I want that again.'

'No, as you say, they can be disorientating, and put you back in touch with experiences and sensations that you have left behind, as it were.'

'Yeah. I'll bear that in mind.' Steve smiled. 'Maybe it was something that I ate?'

'Well, something may have triggered it, something you ate, or saw a picture of, or saw on TV, maybe, I don't know.'

'Well, I can't think of anything specific.' Steve shook his head, aware of just how vivid the dream had been. He lapsed into silence. John sat with him, waiting for him to continue, uncertain as to in what direction Steve would want to take the session. Steve brought the session back to his past, mixed grill had been a particular favourite of his as a child – at least, he liked lots of things, but he used to go to a pub with his parents that did a real 'belly-buster', as Steve called it. Could it be that, childhood favourites coming to mind?

'One thing all of this has taught me is that as adults we are never really that far away from our childhood, whatever we might think, and however much we might have forgotten, it is there, with us.'

John nodded, 'like we never get away from our childhoods?'

'Or they never get away from us!' He paused. 'And yet, we can change. It's not easy, but we can. I've changed. I've gone back to the past and begun to see things differently – then and now.'

'Mhmm.'

'But it's not easy, and I can understand people not wanting to do it, but I know, I just know, that trying to do something about my weight without what we've talked about, it wouldn't have worked. I've needed this greater self-awareness, self-understanding, whatever you call it, to deal with it all.'

'Changing your eating habits wouldn't have happened, or might have happened but wouldn't have been maintained?'

'Either, both, I don't know. But I don't see how I could have changed without changing on the inside, you know what I mean?'

'I do see what you mean, and it's encouraging for me to hear that. Some people do change behaviours without this kind of process – maybe they've already changed inside and the outer change of eating pattern is the final step – maybe. I don't know. We need more research. I'm sure people do. But not everyone.'

'I guess I could have lost more weight more quickly in other ways, maybe, I don't know. But this feels right for me.'

'And I guess that's what matters, that you find a way that's right for you, and that choices are available.'

The session moved on to Steve saying more about how he had changed to wanting to be a father, and he was quite emotional as he talked. It had become something very close to his heart. John didn't comment but acknowledged to himself his sense of the contrast between Steve, bullied at school, finding his own power and becoming the bully himself, spitting out his anger in violence at football matches, then settling down with Jackie, but eating to deal with his inner discomforts and conflicts, and now, now sitting tearfully describing his hopes to be a dad. For John, everything that he had offered to Steve took on a fresh meaning and purpose, the possibility of new life, and of a new life in our life. He felt tearful himself, and did not hold back from letting Steve see how affected he was. It was a poignant moment for them both. Another turning point, or stepping stone, in their therapeutic relationship, client to counsellor, man to man, person to person – and maybe, most importantly of all, heart to heart.

Points for discussion

- What are the main characteristics of change that you have seen evidenced through Steve's counselling experience with John? Relate this to Rogers' seven stages of constructive personality change.
- What are your feelings now towards Steve, and the level of your optimism/pessimism for the future?
- As a father to be, what issues might now arise that might put Steve's altered lifestyle and eating pattern at risk?
- Critically evaluate John as a counsellor, relating your conclusions to his effectiveness in offering the therapeutic conditions.
- How would you relate the content of this session to the processes of change described in Appendices 1 and 2?
- Write notes for this session.

Reflections . . .

John's reflections – 'I feel as though I have been making steadily deepening connections with Steve, as he has made steadily deepening connections with himself. He has changed, and it is a real joy to see. It's not just his appearance, he really is loosening up and becoming more open to experience. He's gone about tackling his eating with a real motivation and, yes, he has had slip ups on the way, of course he has, people do, but he's kept at it. And he has developed a real language for describing his own experiences. He is very much a presence in the room, a person in process. Or should I say a process in person?

'For me, I feel good about the relationship. I get a sense of satisfaction from our sessions. I've learned a lot, and I've enjoyed exploring the process in supervision. I know there is further to go. I don't know how many more sessions we will have, but I look forward to them, as a therapist, and I have to say as a person. I'm still working on the overlap; maybe one day I'll have more clarity around that though I am beginning to suspect that that may never quite be the case.

'I think that counselling people for obesity issues is timely and necessary though may take a while to be accepted within the culture. There is too much lampooning of people with issues of being overweight. It can be funny for the thin people watching this on TV or at the cinema, but how does the overweight person feel? My attitude has changed since working in this area. I have seen too much pain and anguish on people's faces, felt their hurt at being bullied and ridiculed to be able to sit comfortably with, what is, an extremely difficult experience for those for whom their overweight bodies are experienced as a problem, or have been a problem to them in the past.

'It seems to me that society has to become a bit more mature. There is a need for greater understanding as to why people overeat and/or put on weight. For some it is genetic and/or linked to metabolism such that they seem to be able to do little about it. Others eat to feel better, driven by all kinds of psychological reasons. Finally, there are those who do not have to overeat, or eat particularly fattening foods, but who choose to: for social conditioning, availability, advertising, all kinds of reasons.

'I just look at the world sometimes, and it may not be a fair thing to say, but people in some parts of the world do eat more than they need, and do eat foods that cause more health and weight problems, whilst elsewhere there is starvation. It seems to me that humanity has an eating disorder, the pattern of eating across the world is disordered.

'Who do we blame: food producers or food consumers? Governments and food standards departments who don't label food accurately enough or promote healthy eating effectively? Let's put blame aside and try to openly and honestly acknowledge that there is a problem. Then we can start to look for solutions. But until there is a consensus that there is a problem it is hard to see a way forward.

'I've slipped out of a counselling role. As a counsellor, I feel for the people who are faced with the struggle to change what may amount to the habit of a lifetime, with a clock ticking against them as their hearts and other organs are put under stress by their excess weight. It is the human tragedy of obesity that must not be lost sight of. The bullying that can take place. The social stigma that people can feel. The people who die young and needlessly.

'So, I am an obesity counsellor. But what do I counsel for? Obesity? Eating disorders? Eating issues? Problem eating? No, I counsel people, people who happen to have issues related to eating and weight. Weight and eating are symptoms. The focus for effective person-centred counselling and psychotherapy will always be on the person.'

Steve's reflections – 'Well I didn't expect anything like my experience of counselling. Here I am, seven months or so on, more than four stone lighter, having changed so much of my life, and looking ahead with thoughts, hopes and ideas that were literally unthinkable when I started my counselling. What can I say? It's been an incredible journey. Horrible at times, so painful, but it is worth it – I can only speak for myself. I know I have further to go, and I will continue.

'I never realised just how linked my eating behaviour had become to so much of my life, my experience, to me. The idea of breaking it down, realising that I eat for reasons, reasons that can be explored, made sense of, and to some degree dissolved, was totally new to me.

'I may not be the same as everyone, but I have been fascinated by the process. I'm sure others may react differently, but it has made me think about who and what I am in a very different way. And I value that and I thank John for making that happen.

'I suppose what stands out for me from the last few months has been a sense of John's commitment to me. He's there, focused, listening, attentive. I know he's listening. He doesn't need to tell me what he's heard me say. I know that when I speak he wants to hear, wants to understand me. It wasn't like that at the start, I didn't know what was happening, just knew I got worse. I couldn't take responsibility, truth is, I hardly knew the meaning of the word.

'The release of emotion has obviously been important, the stuff that has gone inside me, but it's only really been helpful, I think, because someone was there. To have had those experiences on my own, well, what would that have achieved? Having someone there, that's what has been important.

'I'm sure I'll always like eating, and I will want to maintain a certain size, though quite what the end result will be I don't know. As I sit here now, the idea of sixteen stone sounds acceptable, but when I get there, who knows? Who knows? It's a journey, a mystery tour, sometimes magical, more often painful. But it feels right and that rightness has grown over the months.

'Our last session, both sitting there with tears in our eyes and lumps in our throats. Yes, start of a new life for me, and the possibility of a new life in my marriage to Jackie. A new life. That's what I have, and whilst in one sense it has arrived, in another sense I guess I'm still in labour! Funny that, hadn't quite thought of it that way, and it makes my counsellor some kind of psychological midwife, I guess. Well, maybe the metaphor works because there is a sense of being born again, not in some religious way, but in a very personal and human way. Yes, I am becoming more of myself, getting to know me, and seeking new experiences that will no doubt have an effect on who I am in the future. It's in my hands. Back to responsibility. Life can be merely a journey from meal to meal, snack to snack – as in many ways it was for me even though I did other things, but they held a specific significance in my days. Or life can take us beyond a pre-occupation with eating. I've learned to choose the latter and I feel hopeful for a more healthy future as a result.'

PART 2

Julia remembers her past

Pamela heard a desperate edge to her client's voice. 'It feels a desperate struggle. There is one part of you wanting you to eat to protect yourself, another part is trying to control what you eat. And in the midst of all this the fact remains that you like eating, it's an enjoyable and satisfying experience.'

Julia took a deep breath. 'So, how can I stop myself from losing control? Just trying not to eat as much isn't going to be enough. I can feel that. Somehow I've got to resolve this inner conflict, try to find or make some kind of peace in myself, whatever that means.'

CHAPTER 7

Setting the scene

Julia has been attending counselling for some three months, originally referring because she was feeling unable to cope with life. She was tired, listless, but at other times quite anxious, particularly in the evenings without really understanding why. She's 25 and has a weight problem. It's not a dramatic problem, but it has become an issue. She weighs around seventeen stone and has been big ever since her late teenage years. Her counsellor, Pamela, works privately from home.

Julia has attended nine sessions so far. In that time she has talked about her difficulties in her life, work issues, and generally feeling that she's isolating herself in many ways. She has friends but she feels as though she is distancing herself from them and she is not sure why. Throughout this period Pamela has been offering Julia space to talk freely and to explore what she is experiencing, listening to what she has to say and conveying warm acceptance and empathy towards her and her experiences.

At first, Julia felt distrustful. She wasn't used to people listening to her, not to her as a young woman. Yes, at work, where she had found her niche, she was used to having people take note of what she said. She worked for an accountancy firm, and had become a very trusted member of the team. But outside of work, she lived in her own flat and didn't socialise a great deal. She didn't go out clubbing, or anything like that, she felt too self-conscious and, anyway, she couldn't wear the kind of clothes that her friends did. She didn't feel right. She had found herself pulling away.

The subject of her weight had come up, but Julia had then avoided focusing on it. She knew how much she weighed and really didn't want to think about it. She found it upset her sometimes. Her weight was very much an effect of the quantity and nature of the food that she ate. And she did eat a lot.

She had begun to experience back problems at work, sitting at her desk. She had been to seek professional advice and, well, her body size was identified as contributing to the problem. It was difficult for her to find a comfortable position and she often found herself having to lean forward, and that was what was causing the strain. It was recommended that she lose weight.

Julia had not mentioned this to Pamela, but her back was getting worse and she was realising she needed to do something. She wasn't sure that she wanted to go to a group, she didn't feel at ease in that kind of environment. She had grown to trust Pamela, though she was still anxious about talking about her weight, knowing how upset she could get in counselling sessions.

Counselling session 10: the client connects with her feelings but is unable to voice them

Julia had come to the session with the intention of telling Pamela about her back problem. It had been worrying her a lot and she wasn't sleeping well at nights. Her mood felt flat. The counselling had lifted it, but now it felt lower again. She didn't like it. She wanted to feel different.

'So, how are things, Julia?'

'Not so good.' Julia felt herself looking down as she spoke. Her back was uncomfortable, felt tight, and her shoulders felt solid.

'Not so good.' Pamela sought to convey her empathy not only through using the words that Julia had spoken, but through her tone of voice.

Julia took a deep breath. 'I've been having back problems for a while now.'

'Is the seat you are in OK?' Pamela immediately felt a need to check out whether the seating position in the counselling room was causing or contributing to the problem. Whilst she knew it was her need to ask this question, she also saw it as a communication of her warm acceptance of Julia. The relationship had developed over recent weeks, it was a little more relaxed than it had been at the start. It had taken a while for Julia to settle into the relationship – that was how Pamela had experienced her. She felt that Julia did appreciate and experience her warmth, but there had also been times when clearly, in her anxiety and self-consciousness, Julia had been believing that no one could feel warmth towards her. For Pamela there was an on-going awareness that this was a sensitive area for Julia.

Julia looked up. 'Yes, yes, that's not the problem.' In fact she knew that at the moment there wasn't any seating that was comfortable for her. The chair in the counselling room was comfortable enough, it was just that whatever position she adopted her back still felt tight and aching.

Pamela nodded her acceptance of what Julia had been saying. She didn't want to question what she was saying, but she did want to let Julia know that if the chair did prove to be a problem she would appreciate knowing so that something could be done about it. 'Ok, but if at some stage it becomes a problem to you, please let me know and we'll see whether we can change it.'

Julia smiled, feeling pleased that Pamela sounded so genuine, and that she would change the chair for her if it was a problem. She felt momentarily special. Almost immediately, though, she felt a counter-reaction which was of the nature of telling her that probably that was what Pamela said to everyone. 'I'm sure I won't need to put you to any trouble.'

Pamela heard the response and smiled warmly. 'No problem, Julia, really I would much rather that you felt comfortable than not. Just let me know.'

Julia nodded. She let the topic go. 'OK, but it's not that the chair is causing a problem. My back has been quite uncomfortable for a while, and at work especially, so they looked at my posture at my desk when I am using the computer.'

Pamela nodded. 'That can be a problem.'

'Well, they told me I'm not sitting very well.'

'So, the way you are sitting at the computer is causing your back to give you discomfort.'

Pamela looked pained as she replied, seeking to convey an appreciation of the difficulty it could pose, and her feeling of sympathy for what Julia was experiencing.

Julia nodded. She knew she'd intended to mention her weight but somehow, now it seemed so much more difficult to actually talk about it.

'So, they've made some suggestions for me to try.' She moved in the chair, seeking to free her back a little as the stiffness was increasing all the time.

Pamela watched Julia's movement and saw the wince of pain on her face as she moved. 'It looks painful for you to move.'

'It is.' Julia swallowed.

Pamela maintained her focus and attention on Julia. She didn't feel an urge to say anything more, but rather to wait and see in what direction Julia wanted to take the session; whether she wanted to say more about her back, or the pain, or maybe something entirely different. She trusted that Julia would say what she felt able to say, and that whatever that was would be right for her in the moment.

Trusting the process of the client and of the therapeutic relationship is at the heart of person-centred therapy. Thorne (1996, p. 139) writes that 'there is trust in the innate resourcefulness of human beings, given the right conditions, to find their own way through life. There is trust that the direction thus found will be positive and creative. There is trust, too, that the process between counsellor and client will in itself provide the primary context of safety and nurture in which the client can face the pain of alienation from his or her true self and move towards a more integrated way of being.'

Julia sat, still trying to free her back a little. Her heart was thumping a little stronger than usual and she felt distinctly uneasy. She wasn't sure what to say next. She hated talking about her weight. She'd rather avoid it, but how could she? It was so obvious and it was causing her problems. She'd been seeing Pamela for some while now and she felt that Pamela listened to her, but she also felt that she was probably only doing so because it was her job to do so. Would she take any interest in her if she, Julia, wasn't paying for the sessions? She did value them, though, and they had helped, her mood had lifted in recent weeks but now she felt as though she was slipping back. She wasn't sleeping well, her back kept her awake. She had tried taking tablets to relax the muscles and reduce the discomfort, but they didn't seem to make much difference.

She did feel as well that Pamela cared, she was warm in her manner. At times it did feel easy to talk to her, whilst at other times the doubts would be more dominant in her thoughts. She did and didn't want to talk about her weight – all at the same time. She pushed the debate inside herself to one side. 'It's something that I guess I will have to get used to. It seems as though they can't do much to help my position at work, so . . .' She felt uncomfortable in herself, and quite emotional. She looked down, not wanting to catch Pamela's eyes. She didn't feel very much like saying anything more. She didn't feel that Pamela would be interested. But then, she was worried about it, worried about whether it would ever get better and what the effect would be on her working life if it didn't. She had wondered, in her worse moments, if it did not improve, would she just have to put up with this pain for the rest of her life? It made it so difficult for her sometimes. She tried to disguise it, she didn't want people's sympathy.

Pamela felt a sudden surge of concern for Julia. She felt concern anyway at times, but this was different, sudden, like she felt a deep sadness, a sense of Julia struggling with something. She seemed distant, somehow, as she sat opposite her. These kind of intense feelings she had felt before with clients, and inevitably they occurred at times of significance. She wasn't sure what was happening for Julia as she sat in her silence. But her sense was that it was something important. She didn't want to break the silence and risk cutting across and perhaps stifling whatever psychological process was occurring for Julia, but she felt she should quietly let her know that she was still there for her.

'I'm hear if there is anything you feel you want to say to me, Julia.' She spoke softly, trying not to disturb what was happening for her.

Pamela's voice seemed quite distant, as though it was somewhere outside of what Julia was dwelling on. The issues associated with her back seemed so great, so impossible to resolve. They'd told her she needed to think seriously about losing weight. But she couldn't do that. She could never do that. She could never feel safe if she did that. But she couldn't explain that, they wouldn't have understood, no one would really understand why she had to maintain her weight.

It had seemed to Pamela that after she had spoken, Julia nodded slightly. She took that to indicate that she had heard. As Pamela continued to sit watching Julia it was as though Julia had become smaller, somehow, there was something about the way she sat, she looked like a child, not in actual size, maybe it was more about her posture, the way she was sitting, her head down, her hands in her lap, her fingers moving, rubbing against each other in what looked like a nervous or agitated manner. She respected the silence and said nothing further.

Julia took a particularly deep breath, and then breathed out again. It seemed to Pamela that she was shaking her head ever so slightly from side to side. 'It makes you shake your head.' She again spoke softly, empathising with the body movement but not wishing to disturb the internal process.

Julia was feeling very scared. It was not new, but as she sat in the silence it had grown. She had talked about her anxieties and stresses before in earlier sessions, which had been really helpful, but she had kept herself away from talking about how scared she felt sometimes. But now, well, now it seemed to be more persistent, and more acute.

'I'm scared, Pamela.' She was still looking down, and spoke quietly.

Pamela heard what Julia had said and sensed from her tone of voice and the fact that she was still looking down that it was not an easy thing for her to have said, but that it was quite a dominant feeling at the present time.

'Scared?' She spoke softly, gently questioning, not wishing to in any way convey a sense of pressure on Julia to say more that she felt ready or able to.

'So many things.'

'So many things you are scared of.'

Julia nodded.

Pamela sought to empathise with what she was hearing through the way that Julia was speaking. 'It sounds like a horrible feeling to have.'

Julia nodded again, and felt her eyes welling up with tears. She didn't want to cry, she didn't want to lose control. She hated the idea of losing control, losing control in anything. She could never, must never, lose that. But the emotions were strong. She felt a tear drop from her left eye.

Pamela noticed the tear as well. She reached over to the tissues, took one and offered it to Julia. It was a way of letting Julia know that she had seen the tear, and that she wanted to respond in a helpful way.

Julia took the tissue, but did not lift it to her face. She felt another tear fall, from her right eye this time.

Pamela continued to sit and wait, aware that she was now sitting a little further forward in her chair, and her focus and attention on Julia was particularly intense. She couldn't reach into Julia to get a sense of what she was experiencing, she had to wait, conveying to Julia that she was present for her, that she was being attentive, listening, feeling warmth for her, whilst being aware of her own reactions and responses to what was occurring.

'They tell me that I have to lose weight.'

Pamela felt herself nodding, and she knew that within herself she was not surprised, but that couldn't be the cause of the distress that Julia was showing her. She had said she was scared. Scared of losing weight? Scared of having to accept that she needed to lose weight? She empathised with what had been said now and previously. 'Being scared is linked to being told that you have to lose weight?'

Julia nodded, still looking down. She felt scared but she also felt strangely numb as well, as if whilst she had those feelings she was also slightly away from them, aware of them, but in a slightly different place. 'They say my posture is not good because of my size.' As she spoke, Julia lifted her head to look at Pamela. She was touched by the look in Pamela's eyes, which she experienced as warm, accepting, sympathetic. Although she, Julia, knew that Pamela did not, could not know, what she, Julia, was experiencing . . . or why.

'Your posture because of your size is causing you the problem?'

'So, if I want my back to improve, I have to lose weight.'

'Mhmm, to improve your back you have to lose some weight.'

Julia shook her head and sighed. 'I can't do that, but I don't want my back to be like this, and maybe get worse.'

'So, what you're saying is that you can't lose weight . . .'

Julia was shaking her head. '. . . no, no, I can't.'

'OK,' Pamela was aware she hadn't finished what she had planned to say. But she focused on Julia's response, 'so what you are clear about is that you cannot lose weight, am I hearing that right?' Pamela felt she needed to be clear as it seemed so important.

'No, I can't lose weight.' She took a deeper breath and sighed again as she breathed out. 'And I don't find it easy to talk about.'

'No, it's not at all easy, it's a very sensitive topic.' Pamela deliberately avoided using the word "issue", it was such a therapy-centred word, and probably not a word that a client would naturally have in mind.

Julia sat with her feelings. She could feel that churning sensation in her stomach, and a feeling of almost faintness. She felt so torn apart. She so wanted to be free of her pain and worries about her back, and so wanted to be like other people, feel confident like they did, wear the fashionable clothes, the size 10s or 12s – realistically she knew she couldn't expect to be less than that, but . . . she dare not, could not, yet so wanted to be like other women her age. She felt so miserable, so worn down by it all. So tired . . .

Pamela sat maintaining her attentiveness. The room felt very silent, her attention seemed to be heightened as she continued to watch and wait, holding her feelings of warmth for Julia in her heart. She felt it was important to maintain this attitude even though she was not, in the moment, able to verbally or visually communicate it.

Warmth or unconditional positive regard is not simply something to be communicated, but is an attitude to be held. It brings the counsellor into a particular heart-centred state, contributing to the climate of warm acceptance in the relationship. It renders the counsellor sensitive – at a heart level – to what is present for the client. It helps to maintain a quality of receptivity.

Whatever the person-centred counsellor seeks to communicate by way of unconditional positive regard, it has to be heartfelt to have true value and meaning, and therefore genuine therapeutic effect.

Julia could feel a familiar sensation in her body, more than being scared, closer to fear, real fear. No, it was more than that, it was closer to the terror that she had experienced in the past and which still haunted her. But she desperately wanted to avoid feeling that now. She hated it and she hated herself. She wished she could just disappear, be invisible. She felt like she wanted to die, that maybe she would be better off dead. What was her life going to be like, now and in the future? How could it ever change, be any different? She couldn't imagine it being different, she could only imagine it getting worse.

Her internal world of fear and anxiety, of hopelessness, was so present, so much in the foreground of her experiencing that she quite lost her awareness of where she was. Her feelings swirled around her, driving her emotions to the surface, which she fought to push away. She simply did not know what to do. She felt utterly wretched – not a new experience – and one that she was in the habit of keeping to herself as she had done all of her life, never daring to say anything. She felt unable to speak now, as though her feelings could not reach her throat, they were locked in her churning stomach and in her swirling head. But her mouth felt firmly shut. She continued to sit. Time passed.

Pamela continued to maintain her focus, she was not aware of what was happening for Julia, only that she now seemed very much in her own thoughts and probably feelings. Clearly, there was a process happening, it wasn't an 'I don't know what to say next' silence, but something deeper, something that was far from empty. Again the nagging question, should she convey to Julia a sense of her presence? Effective therapy required a minimal degree of psychological contact. If she left Julia where she was in herself, was that contact lost and, therefore, the therapeutic alliance temporarily broken and, if so, what effect would that have on the process? Indeed, would it stop being a therapeutic process? She decided she needed to convey her empathy for what was being communicated and her warm acceptance of Julia as a person.

'You're very much in your thoughts and feelings, Julia, and if you want to talk to me about what is happening, I am here and I want to help.' She spoke from the heart, from a genuine desire to reach out and help her client.

Julia heard Pamela's voice, again it sounded distant. '. . . I am here and I want to help.' The words sounded real, they touched something within her, a part of her that so wanted someone, anyone, to be there for her. It was that part which now responded, driving emotions to the surface that Julia simply could not contain, that broke through the barrier inside herself that she had been desperately shoring up. She started to sob, her shoulder jolting up and down, each jolt causing the ache in her back to feel more present. She couldn't hold back the tears any more and she felt herself going weak. She wanted to slump down. Her breathing came in short breaths. She swallowed and began to regain control over her tears. She took a tissue and dabbed at her eyes.

'Sorry.'

'You feel sorry for crying?'

Julia shook her head. No, she didn't feel sorry for crying, it was one of those automatic things you said when you cried, when your emotions got the better of you. She'd said something wrong. She shouldn't have said sorry. She felt she was being judged, criticised, she shouldn't have felt sorry. She felt herself closing down, she wasn't sure that she wanted to say anything more.

The counsellor has gone beyond empathy and warmth for her client, and given that this is a client who has low self-esteem and anxiety, she is more likely to need reassurance with an 'it's OK to cry' response.

> The risk is that now, rather than the part of Julia that has forced itself to the forefront of her experience in response to what Pamela said previously remaining in control, the part of her that carries her self-doubt will now emerge and may block any further release of emotion.

'I'm OK.'

Pamela could see that clearly Julia was not OK. Yet she obviously needed to convey to her that she was. She could only assume that, for whatever reason, Julia was unable to trust her in this moment with the depth of her 'not OKness'. But to comment on that would be to push, and to make an assumption. Yet Pamela felt strongly that Julia was not OK and she, Pamela, did not feel OK with letting it go.

> An interesting predicament – the client is not OK but says that she is; the counsellor feels distinctly not OK about not saying what she is sensing to be the client's experience. Should the counsellor accept her client's need to convey what she has, or confront it? Should her empathy towards what the client has communicated be the primary factor, or should the counsellor be congruent to her own experiencing, and voice it? And how does her warm acceptance of her client impact on shaping her decision as to how to respond?

Pamela kept her focus on her empathy. She tried to keep to a view that when in doubt, empathy first. The client was communicating what she needed to, and that must be received, and the client needed to know that. And she had to maintain her heartfelt warmth, hoping that, when she felt able, the client would communicate more and maybe indicate that she was not OK.

'You're feeling OK.' Pamela voiced it as an empathic statement rather than as a question. Julia had spoken in that tone and she wished to empathise with that.

Julia felt herself responding inside herself with a contradictory internal dialogue of 'no I'm not, yes you are'. She said nothing, aware of the two voices inside herself. She knew that the truth was that she wasn't OK. She knew that, but she rarely ever admitted that to anyone, only occasionally to a friend, but never going into lots of detail. She found it hard to trust people. She wanted to, oh how she wanted to, wanted to feel that she had a real friend, but she didn't, and she wasn't sure that she ever could or would have that kind of friend. Yes, she had friends, but, well, she never really talked about her problems, her worries, not the really deep anxieties and fears, only the more day-to-day ones. That always felt safer but never felt really satisfying.

She shook her head. The words wouldn't come out, somehow they remained blocked in her throat and her mouth remained firmly shut. She had closed her eyes. She didn't look up.

Pamela saw Julia's head movement. She guessed that it was hard for Julia to voice it, but her head movement was saying enough. She knew it was important to respond carefully, sensitively and genuinely, and without hesitation.

'You're not OK, but it's so hard to say it.'

Julia nodded, her eyes still closed, her head still down.

Pamela felt she needed to keep in contact, maintain communication with Julia.

'Things you want to say, but . . .' Pamela deliberately left the sentence unfinished and the truth was, she didn't know how to finish it.

Julia slowly lifted her head as she took a deep breath, her mouth still clamped tightly shut. She slowly opened her eyes, they were still full of tears. Pamela watched her movements. She felt her own heart go out to her, it was a very human moment. She did not know what Julia was unable to tell her, and perhaps, in the moment, she didn't need to know. This was a therapeutic moment that went beyond words, and Pamela knew that her facial expression, what was in her own eyes, was going to count for so much. And she knew she couldn't try and make herself be a particular way. It was a moment for utter genuineness, a moment for two human beings to reach out to each other in some unseen, unvoiced manner – therapy beyond words. It was in the eyes – mirrors of the soul – where genuine unconditional positive regard could be seen. She knew she felt warmth for Julia, she trusted herself that she was communicating this. Yes, she felt sympathy as well, sympathy for a woman who was in deep pain and anguish.

Julia looked deeply into Pamela's eyes, searching, trying to know whether she could be trusted. She saw caring in her eyes, she saw something in her face – she wasn't able to give it a name – but it had a soft quality, yes, softness, that was what it was. It wasn't like so many of the faces she saw – hard, and cold. This face seemed warm. She felt strangely a little more at ease in herself.

Pamela felt Julia reaching out and looking into her eyes. She returned the eye contact. She trusted the process. What was happening needed to happen. No need to say anything, no need to behave in any way that would distract her client from what she needed to do.

The person-centred counsellor will want to trust what is occurring within the client and the therapeutic relationship. She may not understand what is happening, but that is not required for it to be trusted. The temptation may be to smile, to physically reach out, to say something, but care must be taken. If a movement is made, or words are spoken, why? The client is reaching out through her eyes. Empathy for this is to respond in a similar manner. It is not for a counsellor to break the contact, but to remain genuinely present, offering what the client needs.

Julia felt a calmness and a kind of reassurance. She didn't want to say anything else. Somehow that need had temporarily passed. She felt she needed time to reflect, to be with what she was now experiencing in herself. She looked away and noticed the time. The session was almost due to end. She felt that she needed to take time to think. There wasn't time to say anything much, anyway. She felt that maybe she could say more now, but that it would have to wait, and maybe that was the right thing anyway.

'Thank you. I need to go and, well, think about things.'

Pamela nodded, aware that she had no idea what these things were, and that in truth she did not need to know what they were.

'Mhmm, it's what you feel you need to do.'

Julia took a deep breath and nodded. 'Yes. It's been a difficult session for me, but I think it has been helpful. But I need time to think.'

Pamela nodded. 'Fine.'

'And I'll see you next week.'

They confirmed the time would be the same and Julia left, still feeling a certain quietness within herself yet aware, too, that the old familiar feelings were no doubt not too far away, but she didn't want to dwell on them, not at the moment, anyway. She wanted to stay with how she felt for a while longer. She headed back home. She was hungry. She needed something quick and easy – she stopped off for a take-away pizza and chips. She didn't enjoy eating it.

Pamela knew that whilst she didn't know exactly what had happened, and certainly not what Julia had been experiencing, she sensed the importance of what had happened in the session. Something had connected between her and Julia, something she could not put words to. But she was a great believer in the power of eye contact, that in the eyes more could be seen than was usually suspected, and more could be conveyed. Yes, she thought, the real person, the 'who I am' is always hidden, veiled though to a degree revealed through my body – mannerisms, facial expression, etc. But the eyes, that is perhaps where a true glimpse can be gained of the person behind the body, the essence that drives the machine, as it were. What had Julia seen? She did not know. But she knew that she was a woman in despair, searching, searching for ...? She could not be sure what exactly. Yes, she could list lots of things that people looked for in another person when they were deeply troubled by something, but what did she see in Julia? Despair and hurt seemed to be the words that had most meaning for her as she continued to reflect on the experience.

She took a deep breath and took out her file, and began to write her brief notes for the session.

Points for discussion

- Critically evaluate Pamela's application of the person-centred approach in this session.
- What were the key moments in the session, and why?
- Would you have responded differently at any time to what Julia was saying, or how she was being? What would be your theoretical reasoning for these different responses?

- Describe Julia in one paragraph from what you have experienced in counselling session 10.
- What are your thoughts about the therapeutic significance of eye contact?
- Write notes for this session.

CHAPTER 8

Counselling session 11: a painful and distressing disclosure

The session had begun, with Julia saying a little about her week and how she had felt calmer after the last session.

'It was not easy for me to speak last week.'

'No, I was aware that you looked as if you had things on your mind but couldn't put them into words.'

'It still doesn't feel very easy.' Julia had spent time since the last session reflecting on her need to talk more openly with Pamela. She was aware of still feeling hesitant, but that wasn't a reason to stay silent. Yes, she had been upset by the previous week's session – not so much afterwards, but at the time it had affected her powerfully. And it had left her thinking differently about her situation. And her back had been bad, she knew she was caught between, what was the phrase? Yes, a rock and a hard place. A rather cold and hard phrase and maybe that wasn't accurate, it didn't sound emotive enough.

'No, not easy at all.' Pamela kept her attention on Julia who was still looking up.

'I'm not sure where to start.'

'Mhmm, sometimes it is best to start with what is in your mind, and sometimes it really doesn't matter.'

Julia nodded and thought for a moment. What she was thinking about now was work, but her thoughts soon took her into the implications and the feelings that she had about everything.

'It's about my weight.'

Pamela nodded. She didn't say anything further. She waited for Julia to continue.

'I have to loose weight if my back is to improve.' Julia spoke with an air of feeling resigned to the fact, but also remaining anxious about it.

'Mhmm, for your back to improve you have to lose weight.'

Julia swallowed. 'And I know they're right. I know that my back problem is because of my size and everything, and it affects my posture at work. They've been really good helping to ensure that my typing position and everything is right, but when I spoke to someone about it they made it clear that the problem is likely to remain if I don't find a way of changing my position. It's me; the desk, chair, screen and keyboard are as they should be.' Julia sat tight-lipped.

'So, they're pretty clear about the link, and that for your back to have a chance of improving, you have to lose some weight.' Pamela was uncertain why this had caused the level of distress shown in the last session, but she guessed there was more to be said.

'Yes, and I know they are right.'

'Mhmm, you can accept that?' Pamela realised she had not empathised with this and appreciated that it was perhaps important for Julia to be sure that she, Pamela, knew that there was an acceptance that the advice was right, hence her need to repeat it.

Julia was shaking her head. 'But I can't.'

'You can't accept it?'

'No, I accept it.'

'But you can't lose weight?'

Julia shook her head again. 'I don't want to lose weight, Pamela, I really don't, I really, really don't.'

Pamela heard the emotion in Julia's words, almost a pleading with her to accept that she couldn't lose weight. 'I can hear the intensity of your feeling, Julia, you really, really, don't want to lose weight.'

'I . . .', Julia hesitated, she didn't know what to say. She felt that she needed to explain herself, but that was what was so difficult. She really wasn't sure what to say, how to say it. Her heart had begun to thump in her chest, and the faintness she felt from the previous session had returned. 'Oh God, this isn't easy.'

'Not easy to tell me about. Take your time. Just take your time.'

The counsellor offers reassurance. She has noted the difficulty that her client is experiencing and out of a genuine positive regard she reminds her that there is no hurry.

Julia nodded and was taking a deep breath. She felt as though the faintness was increasing and her heart was thumping even more wildly than before. She swallowed, 'I don't feel too good.'

Pamela reached over for the glass of water and picked it up, handing it to Julia. She took it. 'Thanks.' She took a sip. Then a little more. She still felt faint.

'I need to lower my head, I'm feeling faint.'

Pamela had watched the colour draining from Julia's face. 'Sure, do what you need to do. If you want to lie down, that's OK.'

'Thanks, no, I'll be OK.' Julia leaned forward. It felt a little easier, but she still felt as though she wasn't in control. She slowly sat back up, her face felt suddenly very cold. She closed her eyes but her head swam even more.

Pamela felt that it was a kind of anxiety attack, Julia's breathing had lost any rhythm, it was short gasps with long gaps between.

'Julia, try and breathe slowly, try to just find your rhythm again.' Pamela mirrored the breathing rhythm.

Julia nodded. She knew what Pamela meant. She tried, it wasn't easy. Once she had breathed out she didn't want to breathe in straight away, but she forced herself to. Slowly the rhythm returned closer to normal although her breaths were not flowing in the normal way, there was still a gasping tone to them.

'Oh God,' Julia blew the air out of her mouth and took another breath, slowly it was easing, and her heart was thumping a little less. 'Ohhh.' She took a few more sips of water. Her mouth had gone very dry.

'Feeling a little easier?'

Julia nodded. 'Yes, thanks. I really lost it then, didn't I?'

'All got a bit too much.'

'I don't know how I can tell you, not if that's going to keep happening.'

'Maybe it won't, maybe it's a reaction and will ease. But I don't want you to feel pushed in any way into saying anything you don't feel you want to say. I really mean that.'

Julia felt the genuineness in what Pamela was saying. 'I know. But I have to say something. I've spent my life avoiding it, but now, well, now it seems that I have to say it.'

This is a sensitive time, the counsellor does not know exactly what her client is struggling to talk about, and she needs to be able to offer a supportive attitude without in any way making the client feel they are going to be pushed beyond what they feel they can bear. The client needs to feel safe, needs to feel that what they are wanting to say will be heard and respected. It is a time for the counsellor to be particularly focused in her work.

The best counsellors are those that handle the critical moments to positive effect. In a sense they are like the big points in tennis, the critical ones that turn matches. These are the ones the best players win. However, as with counselling, these moments only arise because of the groundwork that has already taken place. The client feels ready and able to disclose because of the experiences they have already had of feeling warmly accepted by the counsellor.

'Something that you have not wanted to say before, but now it feels like it has to be said.'

Julia nodded again. 'I still don't know where to start.' She thought about it. The idea of going over everything felt too much. She needed to maybe just say it, get it out – it almost felt like she needed to throw it up, sick it out of herself. She felt herself feeling a little faint again. She had to just say it, it was the only way.

'I was sexually abused.'

The words hung in the air. Julia did not know whether she wanted to look at Pamela or look away. Part of her wanted her to lower her head in some kind of shame for what had happened, another part of her so wanted to see Pamela's reaction. She needed to know, to see, how Pamela would react. And she was so, so afraid of not being believed. She looked at Pamela, who returned her eye contact, her eyes slightly watery. There was a sense of compassion in the look that she saw, she felt heard.

'That's such a difficult thing to share with someone else, Julia. It takes courage.'

'Desperation.'

'Sure, desperation.'

Julia's heart was still pounding but the faintness had lessened slightly. 'I put on weight to make myself unattractive.'

Pamela nodded, she well appreciated what Julia was saying. It was not a new experience for her to hear, she was not surprised, and she knew that Julia's experience was unique to her and that whatever she, Pamela, had heard from other clients, she needed to be sure she heard and empathised with Julia's painful and devastating experience.

'Make yourself unattractive to keep yourself safe?'

'Keeping attention away from me.'

Pamela nodded again, aware that she had a lump in her own throat. These were emotional issues and as a woman, whilst she had not herself been a target for sexual abuse, she knew how women's lives – and she was aware that it devastated men's lives as well who were targets for sexual abuse – how their lives could be blighted by such experiences.

'Yeah, keeping attention away from you.' Pamela kept her empathy very close to the words that Julia was using.

'I was twelve when it started. It was where we used to live, we moved away when I was fourteen – thank God we did.'

'So, it started when you were twelve and it happened where you used to live before you moved two years later.'

Julia felt herself drifting back into her memories, memories that were often around but which she had learned over the years to push away. They could be so vivid.

'I had a friend at school, Hannah, and they lived next door.' Julia took a deep breath before continuing. 'She had two brothers. They were a little older, thirteen and fifteen. I didn't like them much, they always seemed a bit creepy. It was them, they used to touch me. At first I thought, you know, it was just a bit of fun, sort of thing that happens. But it became worse.' She stopped speaking, re-living in her mind – and it felt in her body – what it had been like all those years ago. 'They were always telling me how pretty I was, and how they were the first ones to touch me and that I'd better get used to it. I didn't like it, except in a way I did, but I didn't as well. It was like what I thought was sort of normal, but I knew it wasn't?'

'You were twelve years old, it was a new experience, you didn't know what was normal, it seemed like a bit of fun, but it wasn't, and it became worse.'

'I couldn't tell anyone. They were friends of my parents, you know. I couldn't tell them. And I, well, Hannah knew, but she seemed to think it was funny. Told me if I didn't like it, well, I should tell them to "fuck off". But I never could. Part of me liked the attention, it gave me some nice feelings, exciting feelings, but I didn't like it as well. I suppose her younger brother, Jake, was OK, I sort of didn't mind him so much, but his older brother, William, he hurt me, and he knew it. I think Jake was bullied by him. I think Hannah was as well.'

Pamela maintained her attention on Julia, feeling compassion for the little girl who had been subject to sexual abuse, who had had such mixed feelings at the time, but who had then felt she needed to protect herself from attention by putting on weight. And for the young woman who was now having to come to terms with the effects of that. 'So whilst you sort of didn't mind Jake, it was William who bullied them all, and who hurt you.'

'I've never forgotten it. I mean, it didn't happen all the time, but it happened enough.'

'Once is one time too many.'

Julia had never thought of it quite like that. She had struggled to know who to blame. She felt it was her fault. She shouldn't have been so pretty. She shouldn't have maybe encouraged Jake. Had she encouraged him? Had she? 'It happened a lot more than once.'

'Yeah. Sorry, maybe my response was unhelpful.'

'No, you're right, once is one time too many. And if it had been only once, well, maybe I'd have felt different, but it didn't and I don't.'

'No, no, it didn't and you don't.'

'So, when they say I have to lose weight, it . . . , well, it's not something I want to do.' Her voice was low and had an edge of helplessness to it.

Pamela nodded. 'No, those experiences have really shaped you.' Pamela hadn't appreciated the meaning that could be attributed to what she had said. It just flowed out as a natural response to what Julia had been saying. It was only after she had said the words that she realised, and she had no idea how they would be received by Julia. She felt she needed to say something, but then that would simply direct Julia to the meaning she saw in her words, a meaning that Julia might not pick up on. So she waited for Julia to respond.

Julia heard Pamela's response. That, she thought, sums it all up in a sentence. 'Yeah. It certainly did.' Julia looked down at herself, and looked up, her lips tight, her face full of sadness.

'I hadn't meant it like that, but realised as soon as I said it what meaning it could have.'

'I'm glad you did. It's hard to hear, but it's so true. It's so true.'

Things can get said which are realised to have different meanings. The person-centred counsellor will be honest and open about it if they are challenged. Very often, though, there is some truth to what has been said and it can be a comment phrased in such a way that it reflects something of the client or of their experience.

It can occur particularly when the counsellor has a real sense of entering their client's inner world. What the counsellor needs to ensure is that they stay open to their experience and not feel in some way constrained by having to be careful about the words they choose to use. This would be incongruent and be likely to induce anxiety in the counsellor which would impact on the flow and quality of the counsellor's empathic responding.

Julia lapsed into a silence. Yes, they had messed up her life, but she had also encouraged it, she was sure of it. In those days she had also worn skimpy clothes. She'd never been as thin as some of the other girls, but she had certainly been able to wear the same clothes that they all did. Now ... now, well, now she certainly didn't, and couldn't.

She felt a wave of emotion, of sadness and despair. 'I feel so messed up by it all.' She felt her eyes watering and did not try to hold back the tears.

'Horrible feelings to have.'

Julia nodded through the tears. 'I-I don't want to feel like this. But I'm scared what will happen if I lose weight.'

'You want to feel different but you feel scared of what would happen if you lost weight.'

'I mean, I know it's silly, I'm older now, but I can't seem to lose the feelings ...' More tears flowed as Julia felt herself to be trapped by her past, unable to be a woman like her friends, needing to maintain her weight, protect herself, keep herself to herself in so many ways. She had to, but she hated to, and she was realising that she was hating it more and more.

'It feels silly but to me it isn't. You feel stuck with feelings from the past that are all too real in the present.'

'And I don't know how to get rid of them. And I can't lose weight if I can't get rid of them.'

'No, it's like they are bound together.'

Julia nodded again, swallowing back the lump that had formed in her throat. 'I can't go on like this, but I'm afraid of how I will be and what will happen. I-I haven't really had much experience apart from what I've told you. I-I don't know how I'd be. I keep away from boys – I mean men ... you see? That's how it is.' Julia sat, remembering times when she had tried to get to know someone she liked, but she had always felt so awkward, and so full of contradictions in herself. She'd wondered about having a relationship with a woman, but she had dismissed that idea, it wasn't her. She knew she was heterosexual, she couldn't change that, but she knew she was damaged, and she didn't want to be. She had feelings for men, of course she did, and yes, she wanted a relationship, she really did, and yet ... another part of her shrunk back from the idea. She could feel it inside her.

'You keep away, and those boys, it's like ...'

'It's like they cut me off, stopped me being who I might have been.' There was sadness in Julia's eyes as she looked at Pamela, a deep, deep sadness as she contemplated what might have been.

'... And that's such a loss.'

'And I can't change what's happened, but I need to change. Otherwise ...' Julia didn't finish her sentence. She knew the end, just more of how it was, crying herself to sleep, trying to make herself believe that it was OK, that how she was for the best. But it wasn't, it couldn't be for the best.

'Otherwise?'

'More of the same.' Julia shook her head. 'I have to lose weight, Pamela, I know I have to, but ...' She took another deep breath. '... but it's going to mean coming to terms with so much, so much that has, as you said, and you were right to say it, so much that has shaped me.'

'And if that is what you want to do, and yes, it does involve coming to terms with what you have experienced and its effect, then it has to be at your pace. No rush. No putting yourself under more pressure than you feel able to handle.'

'I guess it all makes it more complicated. I mean, some people just eat too much out of habit. I guess for them they just have to learn to eat differently and eat less. But for me, well, I mean, what I eat is what protects me.'

'Yes, and you don't want to lose that protection.'

'But I have to, I have to, so I guess I need another kind of protection – eventually. I mean, that would make sense?'

'Some kind of substitute protection?'

'Oh I don't know. I'm not sure what I'm saying.'

Perhaps using the phrase 'substitute protection' is unhelpful. Previously the client was talking quite passionately, recognising she needed another kind of protection. A simpler empathic response might have been more helpful; 'another kind of protection would make sense'. The client would have been more effectively held on the meaning of her own words rather than being perhaps caught in trying to grasp the meaning of those chosen by the counsellor.

Pamela had noted that the session was soon to end. 'It can feel a bit overwhelming, but there is something in what you are saying.'

'I need to think about my diet, and maybe that's something I can talk about here. I don't think going anywhere else people would understand. I feel like I've told you and, well, I'm not sure I want to tell anyone else.'

'We can look at eating patterns, that's not a problem. And, yes, being aware of what your eating is linked to, we can maybe look at that in tandem, as it were.'

Julia smiled and felt tears welling up in her eyes. 'This feels such a relief. I've dreaded the idea of ever talking about any of this, but somehow though it's not been easy, I do feel better for it.'

'I can only say that I appreciate the struggle you've had, and I'm glad that you feel a little easier now that you have told me.'

The session ended with a little more dialogue and Julia left, somehow feeling a stronger resolve to make changes to and in her life. She wasn't sure how she would do this, but she knew she needed to think differently about food, about eating, about her weight. Yes, she felt anxious thinking about it, but she knew she felt different after that session. She hoped it would last.

For Pamela there was a sense of déjà-vu. She had experienced other clients with a similar dilemma. She felt positive and optimistic. She knew it would probably not be easy for Julia, she had a lot of changes to make. And she also knew how, for many people, when they experienced some kind of intense emotional or physical event that had some degree of traumatic effect on the emotions of the person, it could almost seem as though they stopped developing, as if part of their nature gets stuck at that age. She had worked with clients whose emotional age to some degree got locked down at the age when they experienced the emotional trauma. As if they were unable to move onwards, or at least, that part of themselves. She thought about the ideas in person-centred theory around 'configuration within self' and 'dissociative identity'. She could see how a part of a person's nature could be generated by the experience and then that part becomes the dominant focus, but because of the traumatic effect it remains where it was, unable to grow and develop. Other parts of the person may grow around it, but that part remains stuck in time, in a certain sense.

For more information on the theme of how 'parts' develop within the structure of self and how to work with them the reader is advised to read Mearns and Thorne (2000) and Warner (2000). Information about working with these psychological states is also included in Bryant-Jefferies (2003a,c).

Points for discussion

- Evaluate Pamela's quality and accuracy in her empathic responding in counselling session 11.
- What did Pamela offer that enabled Julia to talk about her past in this session?
- How did you react, emotionally, to what was disclosed? If you were the counsellor, how would you deal with your emotional reaction?
- What are your thoughts about 'parts' developing within the structure of self?
- What would you be considering taking to take to supervision if you were Pamela, and why?
- Write notes for this session.

Counselling session 12: ideas for change begin to take shape

Whilst Julia had felt some relief from disclosing something of her experience of sexual abuse, she hadn't really made much impact on her eating pattern. She'd made up her own mind that she would try and cut out fatty foods, and switch to using olive oil when she did fry anything. She had also decided that she needed to cut down on the junk food that she knew she found all too easy to drift towards. Her cooking skills were somewhat limited, she knew that, and she thought that maybe she should do something about it. It had been all too easy since leaving home to buy processed, ready-made meals. But she knew that was bad news, more so recently with a lot of media attention on what was healthy to eat. But she found it very difficult, and on days when she seemed to reduce the fatty or junk food, she found herself eating more sweet things; cakes and chocolate in particular. It all seemed a bit haphazard and she was feeling somewhat dispirited as she arrived for her counselling session.

As she sat in the counselling room the surroundings reminded her of the past session in quite a vivid way. She heard Pamela ask her how she wanted to use the time and she responded by making reference to the previous week.

'Last week, what I was talking about, I really, really hadn't said that to anyone else. I wasn't sure how anyone would react, or how you would react, but I knew I had to tell someone, and, well, it was a real struggle to get the words out.'

'Yes, it was, and you did manage to. And I feel – I don't know what the word is – privileged, to have been the person you told. And I felt somewhat humbled as well, knowing that it is something you have carried locked up for so long. I wanted to acknowledge that.' Pamela smiled as she finished talking, yes, it had been a humbling experience, and a privilege. But she didn't want what she was saying to sound somehow patronising. Julia had disclosed a horrible experience and she, Pamela, had been the person who was told. Yes, OK, that's what she was paid for, but clients had a choice, and some would choose not to disclose such an experience. Julia had made no mention of it for ten sessions, and she would have had her reasons for that, but last week, whatever was happening for Julia, or between them in the session, made it possible for her to disclose what she had kept a secret for so many years.

'I just knew I had to explain why I couldn't lose weight. I knew I had to tell you once I started, otherwise, well, nothing would have made sense. I wanted you to understand. I wanted someone else to know, someone who I felt would, well, I suppose believe me. I never felt anyone would believe me.'

'No, that often happens and it was your experience as well; I can't tell anyone, they won't believe me.'

'But you do?'

'Yes.' Pamela responded immediately and firmly.

The session is beginning with a process of checking out by the client in relation to what happened last week. She is seeking confirmation that she had been believed. Perhaps in the days that had followed she had begun to doubt whether her counsellor believed her.

It is of course quite usual for clients to reflect on issues between sessions and to then come to the next session presenting with a different perception than the one they had previously, or with something troubling them. Having said what she needed to say, and heard the response from her counsellor that she needed, the client is able to move on.

Julia nodded, breathing deeply as she did so. 'I was convinced that by putting on weight I would make sure nothing like that ever happened again. They kept telling me how pretty I was, how I'd have all the boys wanting to be with me, wanting to fuck me. Sorry.' Julia felt suddenly very embarrassed at her use of language.

'That's OK, that's what they said, and it frightened you.'

'It did. I didn't want that, not if it meant boys like William. I really didn't want that. So I decided I'd make sure I wasn't attractive. I ate and didn't try to look pretty. It sort of worked, but it left me quite isolated later on, and people look at you, and you see what they are thinking, it's in their eyes. They don't have to stare, but some do. And I hate it. I don't want that.' Julia felt her sadness welling up again but she was determined not to dissolve into tears. She wanted to try and work out what to do. She'd cried enough on her own, she wanted to work out what to do.

'So, putting on weight worked a bit, but you then got attention because of your size.'

'Because I got fat.'

'Mhmm, because you got fat.' Pamela used Julia's language. It wasn't a word she would have introduced, she felt language was so important and she needed Julia to guide her as to the language she wanted to use.

'I mean, I know I've talked in the past about school, and how it was OK – which it was, most of the time – but I did get comments by the time I was 16, and certainly when I was in the sixth form. But at least it kept the boys away from me, and that was what I wanted, at least, I did but I didn't. I mean, I thought about it but I couldn't, I didn't want to, but I did as well. Oh, I'm not making much sense.' She felt embarrassed again.

Pamela chose her response carefully and sensitively, she could see that Julia was looking a bit flustered as she tried to make sense of how she had felt and what she had thought. 'Mixed feelings, part of you wanting to keep boys away from you, another part of you wanting to be a 16 year old girl with all the usual hormonal impulses.'

'Pretty much. But the eating got out of control and, well, now I've got a problem with that, and I really wonder now if I can change.'

'You want to change, but the eating got out of control and you now wonder whether you can.'

'Life seems to be passing me by. I'm going to miss out on so much. And that makes me feel miserable.'

'The feeling of missing out makes you miserable.'

Julia nodded, only too aware that she usually ate sweet things when she was miserable, seemed to give her a boost, somehow.

'So, what do I do?'

'Mhmm, what to do, and maybe where to begin?' Pamela added the second comment. It wasn't an empathic response to what Julia had said, but felt to her to capture an aspect of the difficulty that Julia was facing.

'I tried to cut back last week, it sort of worked, but I think I ended up eating more sweet things. I certainly haven't lost any weight.'

'Mhmm, so you set out to cut back on certain foods, yes, but the sugar intake went up?'

Julia explained how she had tried to cut back on the junk food but she hadn't really made it stick, and she felt bad about that, and that had probably made her turn to the chocolate.

'So maybe it is about setting yourself targets you can achieve, rather than ones that you find difficult, don't make, feel miserable, eat chocolate and then feel more miserable?' Pamela was trying to capture the sense of what Julia was struggling with whilst also offering some encouragement by embedding it within a constructive idea.

'That would help, I think, but what I think is realistic might not be enough to make a difference.'

'So, you want to make a difference quickly?'

'Well, yes, but not if it means I don't manage it. It's like I go on mini binges throughout the week. I don't really pig out, but I keep nibbling at things.'

'You don't have major binges, but it's more of a constant nibbling away at things, particularly sweet things?'

'It's so easy to just pick up a chocolate bar, have a piece of cake, eat biscuits, anything like that.'

'And they are easy because . . . ?'

'I suppose because I don't have to do very much, just unwrap them or open the biscuit tin.'

'There is something about how easy they are to access?'

Julia nodded. 'So do you think it would help if they weren't so accessible?'

'What do you have in mind?'

'Well, I mean, if I didn't have so many sweet things in my flat. If I tried to not buy them, that's the problem, isn't it? I suppose I might go out, but it would be unlikely in the evening. If it wasn't there. But it's so easy when you go shopping. There's always something that you haven't tried, or something on offer that you know you really like.'

'That's what supermarkets do, tempt you to buy.'

'I guess so. I hadn't thought of it quite like that.'

Pamela was aware that she had stepped away from being empathic, and that it was her stuff. She watched herself get caught time and time again, tempted to buy what she hadn't planned to get, didn't really need, but somehow the idea of having it was the appeal. Often it didn't match her expectation, so many foods were over-salted, over-sugared, and . . . her thoughts drifted to the rubbish tomatoes devoid of flavour unless you bought 'vine-ripened' ones. For God's sake, tomatoes are supposed to ripen on the vine, that's the way nature designed them; not for it to be something special you pay more for. She despaired at the blandness in so much fruit and vegetables. And the different kinds of potatoes – salad potatoes, baby potatoes, roasting potatoes, baking potatoes – all with one thing in common no flavour, no earthy potato flavour.

'Sorry, my stuff, but you're right, if you didn't have sweet things in the home . . .' Pamela sought to bring the focus back to where she had inadvertently steered it away from.

'I have to try and be more disciplined when I go shopping, or maybe shop somewhere else, where there's less temptation, perhaps?'

'Mhmm, any thoughts on that?'

'Less choice in the smaller shops. That might help. I guess I could go to the grocer's and butcher's shop in town a little more. I do go in there for some things, maybe I need to think about other things as well.'

'OK, so shop in smaller shops to perhaps reduce temptation, and try the grocer's and other shops a little more.'

'Trouble is right near it is that really good fish and chip shop. It won't be easy to pass that when I'm feeling hungry.'

'So, the thought of walking past and not stopping at the fish and chip shop feels difficult?'

'Yes, but I think it's not just fatty foods and junk food. I mean, well, it's the sweet things and, well, I do like ice-cream.'

'Mhmm, you eat a lot of ice-cream.'

Julia nodded, and felt rather ashamed as she thought about the litres she got through in a week.

'Well, bearing in mind you aren't going to change everything at once, what can you see yourself changing?'

'I won't stop the ice-cream.'

'Mhmm, OK, that has to continue, same amount?'

'No, maybe I could try less.'

'Could eat less.'

'Hmm, yes.' Julia paused. 'I like the quality ones, you know, I have a 500 millilitre tub most evenings.'

'Quality ice-cream.'

'I suppose I could try and cut it out a couple of times a week, maybe? But then I'd probably have an extra bar of chocolate or something.'

'Mhmm, you'd probably replace it with something else that's in your flat.'

'Hmm, that's it though, isn't it, if it wasn't in my flat, what then? I don't think I'd go out. But I'd eat something.'

'You'd eat something, and what other options might you have for something to eat that's healthy for you?'

Julia wasn't sure what she could eat. 'I don't know, I've never really tried to eat anything else.'

'Never really experienced eating anything else – ice-cream, or chocolate, or whatever else happens to be available.'

'Pretty much. Hopeless case, aren't I?' Julia looked down. She did feel hopeless. She couldn't see what she could do.

'You feel a hopeless case?'

Julia nodded, 'I do. Everything . . . , there's always something else to eat. I have to stop bringing it into the flat, that has to be the place to start.'

'OK, that sounds positive and realistic. And you've said about altering your shopping.'

'And there's the fish and chip shop. I go in there two, maybe three times a week.'

'Mhmm.'

'It's just so easy to drop in.'

'Convenient, yes? Easy to drop in?'

'Yes, some days, well, I suppose some days it's more of a habit, I suppose.'

'Some days it's become a habit to drop in at the fish and chip shop.'

'Fridays. Especially Fridays. I always go in on a Friday. End of the week and on my way home. Guess it's become a habit, except when I meet up with friends, which I do sometimes after work.'

'Mhmm, Fridays are more of a habit.'

A counsellor might have been tempted to have said something like 'OK, so, suppose you only had fish and chips there on a Friday', trying to offer a solution. However, to have done so would have been to have stepped away from a person-centred way of working, and taken away from the client an opportunity for her to come up with her own solution to the difficulty of the fish and chip shop.

'So, I guess that would be the hardest day not to go in. But I think I do have to stop, don't I? Maybe only go in on Fridays and cut out the other days which tend to be any day really, when they're open.'

'Friday seems the hardest day to change, so stop the fish and chips on other days?'

'Yes. Except that when I meet up with friends on a Friday it would mean some weeks I'd go without.'

'You wouldn't want that?' Pamela responded to the tone of Julia's voice and the look of discomfort on her face at the thought of a week without fish and chips.

Julia shook her head. 'But maybe on those weeks I could choose another night.'

'Have fish and chips on another evening?'

'I can try that. It would be a start.'

'Mhmm.'

'What about sweet things, though?' Julia could see how difficult that could be as well. 'It's going to be really hard not to have anything in the flat.'

'Chocolate, cakes, ice-cream, you mean?'

'Yes. I need something else I can nibble at.'

'Something else to replace the sweet things.'

'I suppose it has to be fruit, doesn't it?' Julia pulled a face. 'I like fruit, but I don't really eat much. I suppose I should, but I get bored. I'd rather have a fruit salad.'

'Tinned?'

Julia nodded. 'I guess I should make my own, shouldn't I?'

'Is that an option?'

'Suppose so.'

Julia thought about it. She wasn't sure, but it seemed worth a go. At least she could put what she wanted in it, but not too much, she'd get bored, but she guessed she could vary it.

'And some tins of fruit come in fruit juice, not syrup, maybe I should get those?'

'Maybe.'

'Hmm, still the ice-cream.'

'Mhmm, still the ice-cream, and maybe you can't change everything at once.'

The counsellor needs to trust the client. The amount of ice-cream she is consuming still concerns Julia. She ignores what the counsellor has said and continues with her focus on her concerns about the ice-cream. The counsellor needs to have noted that she sought to reassure the client about not needing to change everything at once rather than empathise with what the client had said. It could be an issue for supervision. She seems to be making an assumption about the client's capacity to change.

'But I know I eat too much of that. I can feel quite sick some nights, but I can't leave a tub half-eaten once I've started.'

'Smaller tubs?'

'Guess so.' Julia felt reluctant to embrace the idea.

'That doesn't sound too appealing.'

'No, but maybe, sometimes, maybe I can try.'

'Mhmm. Maybe you can try.'

Julia thought for a moment. 'I need to make sure I have a shopping list, and really try and stick to it.'

'You feel it would help to have and to stick to a shopping list?'

Julia nodded. 'I have to list the healthy things. I have to try and not buy junk food and sweet things.' She sighed.

'Makes you sigh talking about it.'

'I need to give myself a treat. That might help.'

'A kind of reward?'

Julia nodded. She'd like to reward herself with a cake, something like that, but that wouldn't be the answer she knew that. 'I suppose I can't reward myself with cake, it would have to be something else.'

Within the context of therapeutic counselling a person-centred counsellor would not be likely to give nutritional advice and information. Their focus would be very much on forming the therapeutic relationship and communicating empathic understanding and unconditional positive regard.

However, a counsellor working specifically with obesity may well have undertaken training specific to that role, and may have specialist knowledge. This might then be offered, or perhaps made available in a leaflet, for instance, offering insight into the calories in the more popular foods. The intention would be to help the client to be informed about their choices. Many people do not have an appreciation of the impact of certain foods, the levels of calories, fats, sugar and salt, and the types of fat, some of which are more damaging to health than others.

'Mhmm, something else.' Pamela wasn't going to make a comment. She sensed that Julia knew what she needed to do, and Pamela wanted to trust her to make her own choices. She knew that there was always a risk when someone was planning changes like this that the counsellor would be too pro-active in making suggestions, and not attentive to what the client was saying, leaving the client with a plan devised by the counsellor in which the client had absolutely no emotional investment. She knew that whatever Julia decided to do it had to be something that she herself owned and felt was realistic and felt that it could begin to make a difference.

Julia decided to think about it later. 'I guess the other side to all of this is monitoring my weight.'

'Is that what you want to do?'

'If I don't lose weight I'll feel depressed.'

'Mhmm.'

'But that's the whole point of all of this, isn't it?'

'Part of it. It's about losing weight, but also about changing diet and eating patterns.'

'Hmm. I could get quite obsessive, keep weighing myself.'

'You think there's a risk of that?'

Julia nodded. 'I don't get on them much these days, I don't want to know.'

'So you keep off them because you don't want to know your weight.'

'Too depressing. And there's that feeling of knowing that, you know, it'll keep attention away from me.'

'Yes, so part of you will feel satisfied with your weight because it keeps attention away, but another part will feel depressed?'

'But I have to reduce it. I either have to stop myself from weighing myself, and maybe depressing myself, or I have to be sure that what I am doing will make me lose weight – except then I'll start to feel vulnerable.' Julia paused, aware of the ache in her back. It reminded her of the reason she was embarking on all of this. 'But I have to lose weight.' She stretched to try and relieve the pressure.

Pamela noted the movement. 'Yes, it's your back that has triggered this process.'

'So I have to do it, and deal with what I feel about it when it happens.'

'You sound quite determined as you say that.'

'I am, I have to be. But it won't be easy, I know it won't be easy.'

'It won't be easy but take it one day at a time. Don't carry the previous day into the next – either feeling miserable because you've eaten something you were trying to avoid, or feeling deserving of a reward because of what you have achieved, or maybe your reward could be something other than food.' Pamela hadn't intended to add the last bit. It was something that they had not considered. Whether she was being directive having said it now, well, she guessed she was. It wasn't that she was telling Julia what to do, rather she was offering an idea. Or was she just trying to justify saying something that was clearly directive and introducing something from her own frame of reference?

'Like a CD, you mean?'

'Maybe.'

'Hmm. That might work. And I could maybe afford that if I was spending less on food.'

'Mhmm.' Pamela left Julia to pursue her own thoughts.

Julia's thoughts had turned to that new Rod Stewart CD, all those old romantic songs. She'd kind of fallen for them, maybe something about her own fantasy life that had never been lived out. Anyway, the idea appealed. She could actually make a list of the CDs she wanted, there were a few that came to mind. She could work her way through her list, and, yes, she'd at least have something to show for it. Whether it would work, she wasn't sure, but it felt like it was worth trying for.

'I like that. I can see that.'

'OK, so, you've come up with a few ideas, shopping lists, rewards, changing where you shop, giving yourself permission to go to the fish and chip shop once a week.'

'And I don't think I'm going to weigh myself. I'm going to put the bathroom scales in the back of the cupboard, at least for now. I don't want to know. I want to focus on these changes. They must make me feel better and I want to build on that.' She hesitated. 'Do you think that's wrong?'

Pamela shook her head. 'I think that if that is what feels right for you, then go for it.' Pamela felt no reason to question it, and she wouldn't have done anyway. It was what her client wanted to do, and why not, maybe for her it could help. There wasn't anything unhealthy either in what she was suggesting. Until she tried it, no one would know. She wanted Julia to build on her own ideas, develop her own confidence in making choices and acting on them. She wanted her to feel in control of this process rather than feel it was something she had to do and that it was being imposed on her by someone else.

The session drew to a close and Julia left feeling that she had something tangible to work towards.

Points for discussion

- Was there anything in particular that struck you about this session?
- How were the core conditions made present within the therapeutic relationship?
- Some of the ideas emerged from the counsellor. Is this appropriate from a person-centred perspective, and if so when? What should a counsellor do with an idea that they feel would be helpful for their client?
- With reference to the processes of change (Appendices 1 and 2), where would you place Julia in relation to her eating pattern?
- What could Pamela usefully take to supervision, and why?
- Write notes for this session.

CHAPTER 9

Supervision: non-directiveness and attitudes towards obesity

'Since I last spoke about Julia (Pamela always used the names of her clients in supervision it made it more real as far as she was concerned) things have developed, and very significantly.'

Eric listened, immediately curious as to what Pamela was going to tell him.

'She's disclosed that she was a target for sexual abuse as a child. She was sexually molested by two boys who lived next door. The disclosure came about because she was having back problems and they advised her at work she needed to lose weight as it was affecting her seat position at her computer. But her weight is linked to her need to make herself less attractive. It's linked to her being told as a child how pretty she was and being taunted about how boys would want her; "want to fuck her" was how she put it. It scared her a lot, and now she's trying to do something about her weight, but is also aware that part of her is scared about what will happen if she does. It's a tough one, but not unusual I know. Everyone thinks people who have a weight problem are simply people who eat too much, and that's it. Why can't there be more focus on the reasons why? I know that for many people, and perhaps an increasing number, it is simply habit-eating out of control, but often it isn't. Often there is a reason or some emotional link to their eating. And invariably it is to do with helping someone "feel better", which can be for a whole host of reasons, as we know.'

Eric was struck by the passion in Pamela's voice. He empathised with her tone, knowing that she would know he was listening. They had worked together for some while and had built a constructive supervisory relationship that had developed into very much a co-professional way of working. 'Your client, and these issues, really touch and affect you, don't they?'

'Yes, they do. It was such a struggle for Julia to tell me, such a struggle. Her heart was thumping, she thought she was going to faint, certainly the colour drained from her face. And she gave me such searching looks, as though she was really trying to get inside me, get behind my eyes, as it were, really be sure about me. And that's after ten sessions or so.'

'Mhmm, ten sessions and really wanting to be sure about you. That feel OK?'

'As you know, she's always been anxious and found it hard to trust people, but I didn't really understand why her esteem was so low until now. I guessed it might be to do with her size, but she hadn't talked about that in the sessions, not until now, anyway. I'd not mentioned it, of course. She clearly hadn't wanted to talk about it. It's one of those things. It may be a problem for a client, but it can take a while to talk about it, particularly when it is linked to something else that is even harder to talk about.'

Eric nodded, aware that Pamela hadn't actually responded to his question. 'So, she has taken a number of sessions to feel ready, or able, to share these difficulties with you.'

'Yes, she has, and you asked about how I felt. Well, part of me in a way would have liked her to have felt able to bring me these issues earlier, but then, who am I to expect that? That's one of the features of being a person-centred counsellor. I don't probe for issues; I don't do a formal assessment asking questions, trying to elicit information. I trust my client to be able to tell me, what they want to tell me, when they feel able to. And I very much value that way of working.'

It is very much a feature of the person-centred approach to trust the client's process, that the client will do or say what they need to, when they need to. This is a very clear way of working and requires a particular attitude in the therapist and an acceptance that the client's own process is essentially trustworthy and will take the client to the place that, for them, is most satisfying. When an issue becomes too uncomfortable to bear, when the client's psychological system can no longer contain and conceal it, then it will break the surface.

In this case, Julia's back has precipitated things. In a sense, if we widen out the definition of the actualising process and think as well in terms of connectivity, perhaps the timing for all that happening has been right for Julia. Life can be like that. Things happen for a reason. Julia's back has become bad at a time when she is already building a therapeutic relationship. She had, before her, an opportunity present to disclose her past experiences and to address the effects they have had on her. It is not for the counsellor to speed up or slow down the process, but to remain that human companion on this part of the client's journey through their life.

'And clearly, the time is right for Julia, at least, life has in a sense conspired to bring these issues to the surface, or rather, make them pressing enough for her to disclose them.'

'And from now it is very much a case of one day, one week at a time. I don't know how she will react to all of this, and how she will manage addressing her weight and what psychological and emotional reactions may occur as she does so. She will process all of this in her own way, and I must be respectful of that, and allow her the time she needs. And she may decide to back away if it all feels too much, and I hope that I can be there for her if that occurs.' Pamela could see Julia sitting in front of her, struggling to talk about what had happened to her. And she was aware that she still only knew a little, Julia had not disclosed lots of details. Maybe she would another time, and maybe not, but that was for Julia to decide what she needed to do. Clients didn't always describe everything that happened, for some it was enough to have disclosed a little detail, enough for them to know that someone else also knew, and that they had listened to them, accepted and believed them.

'So, one day at a time for Julia, one session at a time for you both.'

'And remain very open to what may happen. I expect we'll move from looking at the effects of the past and her experience of sexual abuse to looking at her eating pattern and what she is doing in the present. We spent the last time looking at options. She had tried to make changes but they hadn't really worked which I think had depressed her a bit. So we made it a little more structured.'

'We made it?'

'Well, that's one of the issues I wanted to discuss. I felt that maybe I was coming up with too many suggestions, but then, well, Julia was struggling, at least, that was how it seemed to me.'

'So she seemed to be struggling, as far as you were concerned.'

'But I didn't check it out and I didn't ask her if she wanted some ideas.'

'OK, so was it a one-way process?'

'No, no, I wouldn't go as far as that. But it's like whenever there is a need to look at changes I find sessions do tend to move into more of a brainstorm-ing style no, that's probably too strong, it wasn't quite like that, but I try to be open to ideas as well as being encouraging of my client. For instance, we talked about rewarding herself for sticking to a healthier shopping list when she was out buying, and to begin with the reward was going to be food. It was me that later, when we were sort of summarising the ideas, said about the reward pos-sibly being something other than food. Julia took that on board and mentioned buying CDs, and she really seemed to own that. So it was like I introduced something – I suppose I directed her towards a wider set of possibilities, and she then chose the idea of a CD – which I hadn't introduced, and I was then supportive and encouraging of her in her idea.'

Eric nodded, and smiled. 'It's a difficult one, isn't it? If we are not careful we can become totally constrained by the notion of being non-directive, and at the same time there do seem to be occasions – and exploring ideas in relation to changing patterns and habits is one – when there may be justification for shar-ing ideas. But I guess the aim is not to be telling our clients what to do.'

'The difficulty is that what we might justify as being an offering of ideas, the client may receive as "my therapist told me to ...".'

'Precisely.'

'Mhmm.' Pamela stopped and thought about it. 'What do we offer, I mean, funda-mentally? We offer a particular type and quality of relationship. We offer a therapeutic process that was very much seen originally as being "non-directive therapy". We seek to be empathic towards our clients and the needs that they communicate. We seek to feel warmth, to be non-judgemental and accepting. We seek to be authentic. We seek to create a relational climate that will promote constructive personality change – and then we debate whether this means growth or something else. But essentially as a person-centred counsellor I am seeking to offer something that will encourage constructive personality change. That's what I do. That is surely the essence of the approach. Yes, theory dictates that there are particular ways of going about this. Ohh, "dictates" is a strong word, isn't it? But that's how it is. If certain qualities and attitudes are present, communicated and received in the therapeutic relationship then there is a likelihood that constructive personality change will occur.'

'Yes. By offering what we offer we are saying that our goal is constructive personality change in our clients.'

'And with a change in personality can come a change in behaviour?'

'Yes.'

'But also, a change in behaviour can promote a change in personality?'

'That would seem reasonable and is certainly what many believe, particularly from a cognitive-behavioural perspective.'

'But as a person-centred practitioner I happen to believe that enabling the client to change if you like organically, as a result of their own process, with minimal interference and direction from outside, is the most effective way of promoting change that is sustainable and constructive.' Pamela thought about what she had just said. 'That's what we offer, a process with, hopefully, minimal interference and direction. A bit like hatching an egg. The hen provides the conditions – warmth and safety – the internal process in the chick does the rest.'

'Nice analogy. Yes, we don't expect the hen to start to open up the egg and analyse what is going on in order to help the process of the chick's development. It simply provides an incubating environment that in turn helps the developmental and hatching process.'

'It's more like we . . . ., hmm, I guess in the analogy we would say that the hen provides the necessary and sufficient conditions for a chick to hatch, so I guess we are providing the necessary and sufficient conditions for, what, people to hatch?' She smiled.

Eric raised his eyebrows, 'maybe, something like that.'

'Except that an egg can be incubated in the absence of the hen, and still hatch.'

'And there may be other ways of providing the conditions that promote constructive personality change.'

'Rogers offered *a* way, not *the* way. I think we can forget this sometimes.'

Pamela thought about Eric's last comment. 'But I'm not here to justify my being with Julia in a way that cuts across the therapeutic conditions that Rogers formulated. The question remains, "how far can a person-centred counsellor go in offering ideas and suggestions that may be relevant to the issue being explored, but which risk the client experiencing a sense of being directed, or being pushed by an external locus of evaluation to them?".'

Rogers wrote about what he termed a 'theory of creativity' in which he discussed the importance of the person developing an 'internal locus of evaluation'(Rogers, 1967, p. 354). In terms of the developmental process, we can be discouraged from trusting our own internal evaluation process towards something we have done, or not done, by being expected to accept the views of others, regardless of whether we agree with them. A fundamentally important aspect of the person-centred approach is the intention to foster, within the client, a stronger reliance on their own internal locus of evaluation, enabling them to trust their own valuing process. The counsellor who constantly tells a client what they should do is providing an external locus of evaluation which would undermine the client seeking to trust and value their own judgements. Rogers indicated that for the creative people very often their creativity primarily must satisfy their process of evaluation, how others receive it is up to them, but they are not driven by the need for external acceptance, their internal satisfaction is enough.

'The client has to learn to trust themselves, feel confident in who they are and what they believe. You said that whilst you opened up the possibility of seeking a reward other than food, you didn't direct your client to anything specific, but when she came up with an idea you supported her in her choice and showed warm acceptance of her idea. I think it is OK to open things up, but not in a way that the client might feel that what they have been thinking is undermined, not good enough, not right. You might have got a reaction of "so, food isn't a good idea, then?" and then it would have been a very different situation.'

'So care is needed, and great sensitivity to the client's process.' Pamela thought for a moment, aware that she still felt she hadn't resolved her question. 'But, well, I guess it is a matter of being aware of what is happening for the client and in the relationship, to know what can be offered. I think it is an area for person-centred counsellors to explore. When does an offered idea become a direction? Probably, depending on the nature of the relationship, and the client's susceptibility to taking on board what others say, it will depend on how actively the counsellor offers ideas. And, of course, they need to emerge from a sense of connection with the client.'

'It's important to reflect on this when it occurs, to check it out, in case we are getting a step ahead of the client, leading them rather than travelling beside them. And maybe, sometimes, we see the hole in the road before they do and, maybe, if we are genuine in our unconditional positive regard, we are going to say, in some therapeutic way, "watch out!".'

The session moved on to an exploration of Pamela's feelings in general towards clients with obesity issues. This had been touched on in an earlier session, but this had been prior to Julia raising the issue. 'I think that a person is free to make choices, but I know I feel sad when someone has to make choices to protect themselves and as a result do themselves damage. I know that being aware of that does affect my perception. If my client simply ate for no other reason than habit, or maybe what I might perceive as "greed", I would probably feel judgemental, if I'm honest with myself, yes, I think I would.'

'Think?'

'OK, know. Yes, you're right.' Pamela paused, because she was also aware that she could have feelings, strong feelings, and yet in engaging with a client they could diminish. She remembered working with a man who enjoyed hunting, and that was something she abhorred, and yet somehow, because she knew him and felt warmth for him as a person, she didn't experience reactions when he made reference to hunting. Not that he made many – maybe she had given off signals to him that impacted on his freedom to talk about that part of his life, but she didn't think so, she'd explored it thoroughly at the time. She mentioned this to Eric.

'So, whilst motivation for weight gain will affect how you feel, so will the actual process of getting to know the person?'

'Yes, but I'm going to have to own that if I see someone on TV stuffing hamburgers in their mouth in a gluttonous way, with their plate stacked up in ways that are simply not necessary, well, yes, I feel judgemental.'

'So maybe more judgemental towards the eating habit?'

'Maybe, but also the person who is doing it. I think it's the type of food as well. I hate junk food, and I think I feel more judgemental towards people choosing to eat unhealthily. I mean, yes, there's so much nowadays promoting healthier diets and still people consume rubbish – well, that's my view – and I do think like in everything, smoking, drinking, careless driving, all these things, people have to take responsibility for their choices.'

'You don't experience a great deal of sympathy.'

'No, I mean, people can make informed choices, unless the person's behaviour is driven by trauma, difficulties, that kind of thing.'

'So, someone who eats junk food to feel better, to avoid attracting attention, that's OK, but someone who just eats it because it's there and they want as much as they can have, that's unacceptable to you.'

'Yes, yes, in a world where people starve, yes it is. That's me. That's my view. But I would hope that I would not allow that to affect my work as a counsellor, and if I suspected that it did, or that it would, then I may need to re-think working with particular clients.'

'That seems to me to be appropriate. And I wonder how many training courses allow students to address their attitudes towards obesity, or towards eating styles, so they are prepared to work with clients who have weight issues?'

'And not everyone's weight problem is an eating problem as well, of course. People suffer obesity from genetic problems and other health conditions as well.'

'That's important to remember. So, what about Julia, your feelings towards her.'

'I really have warmed to her. I was just so struck, affected, by her struggle to disclose her having been abused, sexually.' Pamela shook her head and took a deep breath. 'Such a struggle to communicate, get it out. I really admire her for it. And I really want to help her. But I mustn't get ahead of her. It's going to be a slow process, I think, and I want her to, well, I suppose give herself a chance of a future that is a break from her past. What it will look like, I don't know, but I think she knows she has to change, and I believe that now she wants to change, it's just going to be tough for her.'

After discussing another of Pamela's clients Eric brought the supervision session to a close as time was getting short.

Counselling session 13: progress is reviewed; the client feels pressurised

The following session began with Julia updating Pamela on what she had achieved with her strategies for changing her eating pattern. She said that she appreciated the fact that there was flexibility, that it wasn't 'all or nothing', as she put it. She could make changes without having to change everything which she could see was simply setting herself up to fail, and to feel bad about failure. She didn't want that.

'So, I have begun to shop differently and, yes, I am finding it helps to control what is in my flat. I'm managing to stick mostly to the shopping list. It's other times, when I'm passing a shop and feel I have to have something, that's hard, and, well, yes, I have weakened sometimes. But I have also begun to switch to more things from the health food shop and the other smaller shops. One thing I'm addressing is jam, trying to get more low-sugar jams. I hadn't realised just how much of normal jams is sugar, never really thought about that much. And I'm looking at the calories, and fat content. Biscuits with chocolate are so much higher.' She looked a little glum. 'But I've found some slimming biscuits, they've got lemon and cranberry ones and they're really quite nice. They also come in separate plastic bags in the packet two at a time, that helps as well.' So I've made some changes, and I am trying to keep away from the junk food, but I realise I need to cook a few more things. I bought a recipe book *Quick Meals for One* – trouble is, the pictures look so good and, well, they make me want to eat something while I look at it! Hopeless case, huh?'

Pamela wasn't going to reinforce her negative judgements but she would let her know that she heard what Julia was saying. 'So, some positive steps, a few slips and feeling hungry when you read the recipe book makes you feel a hopeless case. How would you contrast this last week with the previous week?'

'Oh, much better. I mean, yes, I'm actually making changes, and I'm sticking to some of them, the previous week, well, no, it got worse rather than better.'

'OK, so overall . . . ?'

'Overall well, yes, I suppose I've done quite well. I don't know that I feel any different. And, well, I've buried the scales at the back of the wardrobe. I'm not going to weigh myself. I've got a jacket I bought a year ago, and it's too tight. I've decided my first goal is to be able to wear it. But I know that, well, I'm going to have to get rid of some clothes and that won't be easy, but I like the idea of being able to wear some of the clothes that I used to wear, and then I know I'll have to throw them out as well. But, well, that's how it will have to be.'

'So, think in terms of what fits as a way of monitoring the effect?'

'And only had fish and chips once, like we said. It was sort of OK because I knew I would have some, actually on Saturday because I went out after work with some of the girls on Friday. Drank a bit too much, but, well, you have to have a laugh, be sociable, you know?'

Pamela smiled, 'that sounds really important for you, have a laugh at the end of the week, a few drinks, bit of social lightness.'

'Yes, but I read that alcohol has a lot of calories as well. Is that right?'

Pamela nodded. 'Yes, it does.' It also shrinks your stomach and can reduce peoples' appetites when they get seriously into heavy drinking, she thought to herself. But she saw no point in mentioning it. Keep the focus on Julia's concern about the calories.

'So I should be cutting back on the booze as well?'

'Feel you need to?'

'Well, I mean, I don't drink every night, but I do like a can or two of lager.'

'Depends on the calorific value of the type of lager you drink.'

'There won't be any pleasures left.'

'That how it feels, all your pleasures are being taken away?'

'Sort of. But they're more than pleasures, like I said, you know, I've had to keep my weight on, it's just that, well, I guess the last two or three years it has increased more and, well, maybe my eating has become more of a habit.'

'More of a habit rather than thinking about it in terms of maintaining or increasing your size?'

'It's like when I stand in the supermarket and there's this argument now in my head. And there have been a couple of times, not in the supermarket, but just in ordinary shops, you know, where I've just bought something to eat – usually chocolate, telling myself I deserve it, that why shouldn't I have it? I'm making changes so I deserve it.' She sighed. 'I guess I'm weak-willed.'

'That how it feels, you feel weak-willed?'

'Well, I mean, I'm not able to do what I'm trying to do, and well, it's about will power, isn't it?'

'Change the habit of half a lifetime in a week?' Pamela wanted to ensure that what Julia was saying was set in the context of the whole experience.

'Well, maybe, but I feel I should be able to just make different choices, just do it.'

'Mhmm, like you can stop doing one thing and do something else, without any pull to continue the way it was?'

'Something like that, yeah, I mean, yeah. It's up to me, after all. It's my body, my choice.' She took a deep breath. 'But it's difficult. I think about food a lot. It's made me realise how much time I spend eating, or at least, when I'm watching TV, listening to music, reading a magazine, stuff like that, there's usually something I'm eating. And to just sit and do something without that, it's hard, it really is.'

Julia was also aware that there was one part of her planned changes that she had not acted on. She'd convinced herself that she was already doing enough, that it could wait till later. It was partly because of what was already in the freezer at home, but she'd bought some more during the week. She knew it wasn't good, but somehow it seemed so difficult to really convince herself. It seemed like it was one thing too many to give up. She wasn't sure why this was the one thing that she was really struggling with, well, she wasn't struggling, that was the truth of it, she was simply maintaining her intake of ice-cream.

'So it's hard to just sit, to just do something without nibbling on something at the same time?'

'I tried a fruit salad, it was OK, but a bit of a fiddle to make. But, yes, it was nice, but I'd hoped it would last at least a couple of days but I ate most of it the same evening. So I can't make large amounts, or I've got to be really strong with myself.'

'So, making too much makes it difficult to control your intake?'

'It just seems like I need to eat. I suppose I haven't really thought about it as much as I am now. And in a way I resent it. I mean, I want to be how I want to be. I don't want to *have* to do things. I don't like being told what to do, not really.'

'Mhmm, you want to make your own choices, be free of what others tell you. You want to live your own life, yes?'

'I do.' She slumped a bit in the chair, 'but people are right as well, I have to change my eating, I know that, I have to lose weight, but I want to do it my way.'

'Yes, do it your way, that's what's important, do it your way, like hiding the scales and using clothes to monitor yourself.'

'And, like, rewarding myself with a CD. I mean, I did reward myself. I figured that although I'd sort of not completely kept to my shopping list, I'd tried, and I was making a start, so I did buy one on Saturday, the one I talked about last week.'

Pamela noticed that the expression on Julia's face was one of looking very pleased with herself with a little bit of 'maybe I shouldn't have, but I did it anyway' in her eyes.

'So, you rewarded yourself for making a start.'

'Do you think I was wrong to do that?'

'Did you feel you had deserved it, it sounds like you did.'

'Yes, I thought so. And I had saved quite a lot.'

'So, you felt good about what you had achieved and you noticed that you had spent less as well.'

Julia was back thinking about the ice-cream. It was the one thing now, sitting here, she regretted. But it had seemed such a right thing to do. Somehow, now, it seemed hard to justify it. She thought about mentioning it to Pamela but she had no idea how she could really justify it, not really. The best she could say was that she hadn't started to address the ice-cream yet, but she also knew that the reality was she really didn't want to. The thought of not having it at all, and she couldn't imagine having a little and leaving the rest for the next day. She'd looked at the smaller tubs but they were relatively much more expensive and they just looked, well, they just looked so small. She could imagine how after a couple of spoonfuls there'd be hardly any left. Not worth it. No, she had decided to continue with what she had been having, until she really had to change. Should she say anything, she thought she probably had to. She had to be honest about things if she was really going to get the most from her counselling. She knew that. She'd disclosed some really difficult things and, well, this wasn't so bad, not really. But she felt she'd be judged.

Pamela sat as Julia sat in silence with a frown on her face. She was clearly deep in thought and Pamela had decided not to interrupt her but wait to see what it was that she was engrossed by.

Julia broke the silence, speaking quite softly. 'I haven't done too well with the ice-cream, though.'

Having felt heard and listened to previously, the client has moved back in her thoughts to the problem of the ice-cream. Having felt good about what she had achieved, she then became aware of her feelings towards what she hadn't achieved, and felt safe enough to disclose this and is then ready to move on to explore what she can do about it.

'The ice-cream has proved difficult to change?'

'I suppose I didn't really try.'

'Mhmm, so you don't feel you really tried with the ice-cream.'

'It was difficult, there were three tubs left in the freezer and, well, once I had finished them I just replaced them. I thought about it, a bit, but decided . . . oh it seems stupid now . . . but I decided to leave the ice-cream for now.'

'So, leave the ice-cream at least for now, and carry on as you were.'

Julia nodded. 'It's well, I mean, I guess some people you know have cocoa or something, and I have ice-cream.'

'You mean like a bed-time drink, but you have ice-cream instead?'

'I eat it in bed. I just do it. I mean, yes, I don't think about it, it's what I do, what I have.'

'So, last thing at night, you sort of round off the day with a tub of ice-cream?'

Julia tightened her lips and shrugged her shoulders, nodding slightly as she did so. 'That's me, crazy, huh?'

'Feels crazy?'

'Don't suppose many people do it.'

'Probably more than you think.' Pamela knew that ice-cream was something that people could get into the habit of eating and, yes, eating ice-cream in bed was a habit that she had known people get into and which could get out of control.

'I wouldn't know what to replace it with. I mean, you know, we talked about smaller tubs but they looked so small and, well, I could see that they just wouldn't last very long. Couple of spoonfuls, you know?'

Pamela nodded and thought of the small tubs, and then thought about what Julia had said. A thought came into her mind, but she was very aware that it was definitely coming from her frame of reference. And she didn't want to push Julia into those smaller tubs unless she really felt, herself, that it was realistic and what she wanted to try.

'Couple of spoonfuls wouldn't be enough?'

Julia nodded. 'Hardly worth it. I like to take my time and really enjoy it. I suppose it's another reward.' She thought back as images from her past came to mind. She could remember how, as a teenager, when her periods started, and they were really difficult and painful, her mother used to give her ice-cream, really nice, quality ice-cream – like the ones she preferred now. And she'd have it in bed, lying down. Somehow those memories seemed very vivid, very present to her as she thought about her room, the bed, the TV, and half lying, half sitting, trying to get comfortable, and having this tub of ice-cream. Small tubs, of course, she'd progressed on to the larger ones much later.

'So, you need more than a couple of spoonfuls, yes, to make it worthwhile.'

'As a child I used to make it last, and I still try to, just love to feel that coldness, and the flavour. I really like the double choco . . .' she hesitated. 'Oh, that's probably the worst one as well, isn't it, all the calories.'

'Probably.' Pamela looked at Julia who had suddenly looked quite pained at what she had just said. 'It's awful, isn't it?'

'Yes, yes it is. But, well, I must do something about it, mustn't I? I mean, I can cut back on other things, but somehow ice-cream, it sort of doesn't feel right to not have it.'

'So much a part of your life, of your nightly routine, you mean?'

Julia nodded. 'But it isn't good, is it, not really?'

'You sound as though you are having to try and convince yourself.'

'No, not really. It's like, well, I mean, it's like I know . . . I know I should stop, but it's like it's what I do. I can't imagine not having it. I mean, sometimes I don't, if I run out and haven't been able to get any, or I'm staying with friends or with my parents, then, well, then it's different I suppose. With friends well it's like a different routine, and the same with my parents, though my mother still has tubs of ice-cream for me. She's never forgotten and it's become a sort of ritual, I suppose, when I visit. She always takes great delight in telling me she has tubs of ice-cream for me.'

'Small ones?' Pamela wasn't sure that she'd said the right thing, but there was something about trying to help Julia to acknowledge that maybe she could get by on a smaller tub.

'Yes, yes, but she gives me a smaller spoon.'

'Mhmm. So, a smaller tub with a smaller spoon.' Pamela didn't want to make any connections for Julia, but she knew she hoped that she would.

'Is that what you think I should try at home?'

Pamela had to smile, she'd obviously responded with a certain tone in her voice, or had a look on her face that had communicated her feelings.

'Just a wonder, I really don't know.'

'Hmm, I know you're probably right but, well, I don't want a smaller tub, I want to have what I like, what I'm used to.'

'Sure, and maybe that's OK too.' Pamela wanted to take any pressure off Julia. She could tell from her tone of voice that she was feeling irritated and that was probably the result of feeling she was being pushed into something she did not want.

'I don't want to talk about the ice-cream any more. I'll do what I can. I'm really not sure I want to change that, not now, not yet. I need my routine. I'll change other things.'

'And I really appreciate hearing your determination. You're going to do it your way and, yes, I want to honour that. Maybe I was being too clever, trying to outwit you on the tubs and the spoons, and I apologise for that. I just want to help, but I have probably overstepped the mark. You know what you want to do, go for it. You're making a start, and maybe what's more important is to make that stick so you can build on it.' Pamela was genuine in what she'd said. She could tell by the level of irritation and the way Julia suddenly wanted to stop talking about the ice-cream that she was feeling pressured. Yes, she had tried to be too clever, without thinking she'd been looking for an opportunity to challenge Julia. She would need to take that to supervision. And she appreciated that Julia had stuck up for what she wanted.

The issue of the ice-cream is deep-seated and it is connected to the client's childhood experiences. It has a lot of added meaning for her. She doesn't want to change, at least, part of her doesn't which has now found a strong voice and is cutting off further discussion, leaving the part of her that knows she has to change it pushed to the background. The counsellor apologises, aware of the sudden change and that it was largely due to what she had said. She could, however, have stayed with the empathy for her client and acknowledged that she didn't want to talk about ice-cream any more, and wasn't sure she wanted to change it. It is not clear what response would have been best. The danger is, however, that the part of the client that has asserted itself might trigger a much larger lapse or relapse of the client's changed eating pattern.

Time was passing and the rest of the session was spent talking about Julia's work at the accountants. It was clear that she really did love her work, and the people she worked with. She said how she felt at home there, that it was a family business although it was quite big as well. She said that they had talked about her doing some further training come the new term in September and they were discussing options with her. She felt that she didn't want to let them down, that they'd been good to her. She wanted to sort herself out and make a real go of it.

After the session Pamela sat and reflected. She had been over-the-top about the ice-cream, and she wondered why. She certainly knew she wanted to explore it in supervision, but she also found it helpful to 'self-supervise', as she called it. A conversation she had overheard in a queue once came back to mind, that some companies put animal fat into the ice-cream. It had put her off and she was now more wary of what she bought. She didn't know if it was true, but it had stayed with her. She'd felt, and to some degree still did when she thought about it, a kind of revulsion at the idea. She wondered how many vegetarians might be unaware, assuming it was true.

How easily we are affected by something that provokes a feeling of dislike for something. She thought of Julia, and how easy it is for our whole lives to be blighted by things that are said to us about something that provokes a strong reaction. Pamela wondered whether she was carrying a kind of 'anti-ice-cream' issue, provoking her to be more pushy towards her client? Was she? She would certainly never have eaten ice-cream like Julia does. She couldn't, wouldn't feel right. Wouldn't feel right. Hmm. Or would she secretly like to? Was there envy? Was there? Surely not. Or was it her problem-solving nature seeing a way for change to happen and being too pushy?

What had been going on for her? Was she trying to prove something to herself, to not be defeated by the one thing that her client was struggling with? Was she almost living out her client's drama, trying to do what her client was finding difficult and eventually saying that she wasn't going to try with? How did that idea fit with person-centred theory? Maybe it was a combination of her own stuff – problem-solving tendency, bit of an anti-ice-cream attitude, concern for her client's well-being and not wanting to be beaten in wanting to help her – all coming together and just tipping her into a more directive attitude. Well, she knew she needed to continue to self-monitor and maybe talking it over with Eric would help when she next saw him.

Points for discussion

- Were there other issues that, had you been Pamela, you would have taken to supervision?
- What are your views on whether a person-centred counsellor should offer suggestions to a client seeking to make changes?
- Whilst the conditions for constructive personality change may be viewed as being 'necessary and sufficient', this does not mean other responses will not be helpful. Discuss this viewpoint.
- How present were the 'core conditions' in counselling session 13? What might have been more present?
- Concerning the issue of Julia feeling pressured by Pamela in counselling session 13, how would you present this in supervision and what outcomes might arise?
- Write notes for this session.

CHAPTER 10

An update on progress

Five weeks have passed. Julia has attended for three sessions and then there was a week without a session as Pamela was away at a conference. During that period Julia has consolidated her changes and has begun to feel a bit of weight loss. The jacket she wants to be able to wear again is now just wearable, though Julia acknowledges that it could feel looser and more comfortable.

She has decided to enrol in a beginner's cookery class. She wants to feel more confident, but it hasn't started yet. Julia has also talked to her mother about what she is doing – although she has not disclosed anything about the sexual abuse to her – and her mother has been very supportive. She has found this particularly encouraging.

During the sessions, Julia has also talked more about the past, about her childhood, and about the sexual abuse. From what she has told Pamela it seems that what happened was sexual molestation and not rape, however, that is not to in any way belittle the effect that it had on Julia. And not so much what she experienced, but the taunting that she had to listen to as well, and the fear of how it would be if she stayed small and pretty. She talked about how she remembered looking at the glamour magazines, all the models, so thin, so attractive, and thinking that she must never be like that. In one session Julia said how she had sort of gone the opposite to maybe how an anorexic would. It hadn't occurred to her not to eat so as not to develop and mature, she accepted that would happen. It was very much more about making sure she didn't attract attention of that kind from boys, or from men now that she was older, though she regretted it now and wanted to change.

Julia was feeling generally pleased, though she was still struggling with the ice-cream. She was down to the small tubs, that was something she had only instigated recently. Pamela had not made any comment about it; she wanted to leave Julia to make her own decisions and to bring it back to the sessions as an issue when she felt she needed to. She realised that her reaction had probably affected Julia's ability to talk openly about it, and she regretted that.

In supervision she had talked it through. Why she had reacted so strongly, she was still unclear. But she was aware that it had happened and, yes, she was putting it down to somehow experiencing a need to be clever, to have answers, to be able to solve what, for her client, at the time felt unsolvable. She knew that she had been a problem-solver by nature before coming into counselling, and that came out of her previous work within a Human Resources Department in the world of business. Her work had been to resolve difficulties and problems with teams and managers. She had reached a point of burn out and had already begun to take an interest in counselling, having started some training. Her own stress took her into therapy and one thing lead to another, and now she was in private practice as a counsellor. And, yes, that problem-solving part of her occasionally came to the fore. Often she noticed it, but sometimes it would trigger a response from her towards her client that sometimes could prove quite helpful, though at other times could be more problematic.

Counselling session 18: the past fights back and clarity emerges

Julia was walking up the path to Pamela's door, reflecting on her day at work. She had come straight from work, usually she dropped in at home to freshen up, but today had been hectic, they had fallen behind on a deadline and it was just one of those days. At least it seemed that it was back under control now. It had meant more typing for her and she had had to do some checking of figures for a report. Her head was still whirling with it all. She felt strangely detached from the counselling process, and felt it likely that it would take her a while to really 'arrive' for the session.

She knocked on the door. Pamela answered and invited her in. She went into the counselling room, taking her usual seat opposite the door, by the window. She looked around. The room was familiar, of course, but she was aware that it felt different. Or maybe it was her, the day still affecting her.

'So, I hope the two weeks have been OK. How do you want to use today?'

'How was the conference?'

'Fine, thank you. All part of my professional development.'

'Yes, I'll be starting my course soon. It's all been agreed. In a way I've probably been doing a lot of it anyway. My real work is secretarial, but I have a good head for figures and they use me to check reports and papers as well. So, it's a diploma and they've said if I want to carry it further they would support me in that. So that feels good, something to look forward to.'

'You're excited by it?'

'Yes, I am. I like figure work and, well, it would be good to really learn more in depth. We did business studies at school, which I think helped me to get the job, although as you know it wasn't my first job. Took me a while to decide that accountancy was the environment I wanted to work in. And the people, of course, I just felt like part of the team so quickly.'

'I get a real sense of your enthusiasm, the job, the people.'

'I like it there and I feel really valued, and that means a lot to me.' Julia felt a little emotional as she came to the end of what she had been saying.

'Yes, yes, I can see that in your eyes.'

'All the other jobs, well, you were just another typist or secretary. I had done temping and that was, well, sometimes it was OK, but sometimes you were like on a conveyer belt, no, you were the conveyer belt, they really worked you hard. And I don't mind that. But it's about attitude. Some people just look down on you all the time, you're just the temp, just the typist, just the secretary. I used to put up with it, thought that was how it was, but I didn't like it. Now, well, now it's really different, and I feel much more relaxed.' Julia moved her shoulders. 'Back still a pain, though. I think it's a little easier. I've been doing some gentle exercises, nothing too strenuous, but some movements to try and make it more supple. And . . .' She paused for dramatic effect.

'And?' Pamela returned a quizzical and curious expression.

'This is the jacket I've been wanting to get into.'

'It fits nicely, and it's certainly not too tight.'

'I know. So, first goal achieved, and it feels good. It's not going to be easy to want to reduce more so that it's too big, but I guess I can wear something thicker under it for a while when that happens, before I have to let it go. But . . .' Julia sat up in the chair, 'it feels good.'

'I'm really pleased. It does look good on you. I can see why you chose it as your first goal.'

'So, now I must lose a little more. And I think I will. I've been doing well. Not without a few slips.' She thought of the cake she'd bought. She knew she didn't need it, but it was one of those moments of weakness. It had been triggered by a man trying to chat her up and it had left her feeling anxious on her way home. She bought it and ate half of it, even though she knew it wasn't the answer, but she couldn't seem to stop herself. She explained what had happened to Pamela.

'So the experience and the anxiety triggered you into eating.'

'I don't know what happened, but it was like I had to eat something, *had* to, there didn't feel like any choice. Does that make sense?'

'That was how it felt, like you simply had to eat.'

'And it had to be something sweet, somehow, no, maybe not sweet, but something fattening, something that would fill me, yes, more about it being bulky. Biscuits wouldn't have done, and I'm not sure that chocolate would.' The pace of her speech increased. 'If I'd been going past the fish and chip shop then probably, maybe, I don't know, I really don't know, but I just didn't feel like I was in control and yet somehow I did because I knew exactly what I was doing.' She paused to take breath. 'What happened to me?'

It is as though the part of Julia that had developed and drove her to eat to avoid being attractive had re-asserted itself, and it clearly now felt like something very different to her as she had been spending the past few weeks distancing herself from it. This can happen as a person tries to establish a new way of being. We can think of it in terms of being elements within the person's structure of self fighting back, or simply as a behavioural reaction to a powerful trigger. It seems strange to Julia because she has not been so firmly identifying with that part of herself for some while, not eating to satisfy that part's need to maintain her size and the set of satisfying feelings that this brings and which this part requires.

From a person-centred perspective we can use the notion of 'configurations within self' to understand this process; each part having its own set of associated thoughts, feelings and behaviours. An experience occurs, in this case the man chatting up Julia, and immediately the part is, in a sense, activated; it comes to the fore bringing with it all that is associated with it. Julia feels and thinks in a particular way and is driven to behave in a particular way – eating food that will maintain or increase her weight. Julia is left confused, for now she has a sense of being someone other than this part.

'So, you found yourself acting in ways, and maybe thinking and feeling too, like you did in the past?'

'I suppose so, but I never really thought about it then. I mean, I was just being me, you know, but this felt like another me, it really did.'

'So, it felt like another you, the you that you were.'

'Yes, yes, like I was back to being who I was, but then, well, I'm not any more, am I?' Julia looked at Pamela, clearly bemused, clearly searching for some kind of answer to make sense of her experience.

'No, you are building a new you.'

'But I'm still the old me as well. I mean, sitting here now, I can feel those old feelings, they feel close and it's like I could slip into them? Talking like this, it brings me closer to them. I can feel myself getting anxious and, and ...' Her voice trailed off.

'And.'

'I've got to eat, I have to. I can't get smaller, I can't, I'll attract men, I can't, I won't, I mustn't.' The agitation in Julia's voice was very apparent. For Pamela it seemed clear that Julia had slipped back into that part of herself that was so vulnerable, so in need of using weight to feel protected. It was a part of Julia that must receive the same quality of empathy and unconditional positive regard, a part that needed to be heard, warmly accepted and understood, the part that had fought to stop her disclosing the abuse, the part that was kept away from people over the years, that kept Julia safe and unattractive, as far as it was concerned.

'You can't, won't, mustn't attract the attention of men.'

'No, no, no I mustn't do that. It will be awful. I can't. I won't know, don't know what to do. I-I ... I must go. I must eat. I'm getting too small. It wouldn't have happened if I hadn't changed things. I must stop. I must protect myself.' Julia's eyes looked slightly wild as she spoke, there was such an intensity to her voice, such conviction that she had to eat the foods that would restore her weight and give her protection. In herself she felt utterly sure of what she was saying, no doubt, no doubt at all.

'You feel as though you are getting too small and that fills you with so much fear. You feel you have to eat to avoid the attention of men.'

Julia heard Pamela speaking, but it was the Julia dominated by the very frightened and vulnerable part of herself. 'Yes, yes, I must. I can't let it happen, not again.'

'You can't let it happen again.'

'They'll make me do things I don't want to do. They will. They told me.'

'They told you?'

Julia nodded still in an agitated way. 'Yes, they told me, Jake and William told me. I hate them but they scare me. I believe them. I hate them. I don't know what to do. I mustn't be attractive. I mustn't.'

'You feel like you must avoid being attractive because of what William and Jake told you.'

'Yes, yes. They told me about what I'd have to do. I-I didn't know.'

'They told you about things you'd have to do, things you didn't know about?'

'Yes, I mean, yes, they said it so horribly, told me I'd be fucked and fucked, and horrible things I'd have to do.'

'They told you that you'd have to be fucked again and again, and do horrible things.'

Julia nodded, the agitation continuing, her eyes still looking a little wild. 'Don't let them do it, please don't let them do it.'

'No, no one's going to let them do it to you, Julia, no one.'

Julia burst into tears, deep sobs, her whole body wracked with convulsions. It lasted for some while, Pamela moved closer. 'I'm going to rub your back, Julia, just gently. Tell me to stop if you want me to.'

A significant exchange, Julia has connected strongly with the feelings and thoughts from her past, and they are suddenly very vivid in the present, generating great anxiety and agitation. It is quite an intense and important moment as Julia as she now is encounters an experience of the feelings from her past. Not only are the feelings distressing, so too is the shock of the split between the two parts of herself. The counsellor offers reassuring physical contact, taking care to say what she is offering before she makes contact. She does not want to impose it on the client, or leave the client feeling that her physical space has been invaded without her having any sense of control.

Julia nodded, and made no move to stop her. Pamela felt she needed to offer human contact, something reassuring. The fear was about what would happen to her physically, it was physically that she felt she needed to convey her warmth. She continued to rub and spoke gently, though she was not sure which part of Julia was now present. She felt that it was probably the new

Julia, the agitation had passed, the emotional release had a different tone to it. 'You've had a shock, Julia, and a big release of emotion. You've experienced what you have been bottling up inside you. It's OK, it's really OK.'

Julia heard Pamela's words, they felt reassuring, and so did the gentle rubbing of her back. 'I-I've never felt anything like that. It was just suddenly there, just . . . I could feel myself going, sort of it crept over me but it was sudden, I knew something was happening and I couldn't do anything about it. Suddenly, suddenly I was, I mean, I wasn't me, but I was.' She took a tissue, wiped her eyes and her face and looked up. Pamela had stopped rubbing her back and was easing back into her chair.

'You jumped between the two me's.'

'I've never felt anything like that. I just had no control, it's no wonder I couldn't stop myself eating that cake.'

'It's powerful, been part of you for many years.'

'And still part of me . . . Oooh!' Julia shivered. 'That's what I'm up against, isn't it? That's what I'm really fighting here.'

Pamela wasn't sure if fighting was the right word but appreciated that was how it felt for Julia.

'Yes, you are fighting against the old behaviours driven by the old fears.'

'But they felt so real, so, so . . . well, now.'

'Yes, very real, very much in the now.'

'How do I fight part of myself? How do I do it?'

'You wonder how you can fight with part of yourself.'

'But I have to fight it, control it, contain it, keep it away.'

'Mhmm, that's how it feels, fight, control, contain, keep it away.'

'But it's part of me, and I don't like it. I don't want to feel like it makes me feel.'

Having acknowledged that the feelings and the urge to eat are part of her, she is then able to talk about how it makes her feel. She is able to step back and own not only what is present from the past, but her feelings towards it in the present. She is not only separating out feelings but also the past and present. As a result she is gaining a more authentic experience. The reality is that there is a past and present although they had become very blurred because the attitudes and behaviours so firmly established and identified with in her adult life are driven by her reaction to the experience of sexual abuse in childhood.

'You don't want to feel that way any more?'

'No, no I don't.' She paused. She felt her perspective shift, she couldn't have described what she experienced, but it was like a realisation had dawned on her. 'But I will, won't I? I mean, it won't just go away, it is a big part of who I am.'

'It feels like it is a big part that won't go away.'

'It feels more like I have to share . . . I don't know what I mean.' Julia thought she knew what she was trying to say, but the words had dried up and the more she tried to think about it the harder it became to regain that sense of what she had been trying to express. 'I've lost it.'

'Mhmm, take your time, don't try too hard to remember.' Pamela tried to help Julia stay with her experience in the hope that she might reconnect with it and express what it was. It somehow felt important. Julia's voice had changed again, suddenly calmer, more reflective, as if she had momentarily stepped out of the battle in some way.

'I can see that there is the me that I was and the me that I am developing. And they're in conflict. And it's all about eating, food, weight; and what's so difficult is the reality that I enjoy eating, you know?'

Pamela nodded. 'Yes, that's part of the difficulty, you enjoy eating.'

'And I can't stop feeling that way. That's my reality in the midst of all this craziness.'

Pamela heard a desperate edge to her client's voice. 'It feels a desperate struggle. There is one part of you wanting you to eat to protect yourself, another part is trying to control what you eat. And in the midst of all this the fact remains that you like eating, it's an enjoyable and satisfying experience.'

Julia took a deep breath. 'So, how can I stop myself from losing control? Just trying not to eat as much isn't going to be enough. I can feel that. Somehow I've got to resolve this inner conflict, try to make some kind of peace in myself, whatever that means.'

'Mhmm, find some way to resolve the conflict, find some kind of peace.'

'It's like I need to reassure myself that it's OK? Like I need to find some way of feeling secure, but I don't know where to find it.'

'Something about not knowing how to find reassurance and security.'

'I knew that anyway, but not so acutely as perhaps now. That's what's different. It's like I really *do* need to feel secure, and that part of me that drives me to eat to put on weight, to I think you said "protect yourself" and that's it, and it gives me a reassuring feeling, that sense of feeling full, that's satisfying as well, and that's sort of the reassuring bit somehow. Does this make sense?'

'Let me say how I am hearing what you are saying, Julia, it's like everything is sharper now, the need for reassurance and security feels more acute, more immediate, more of an imperative, perhaps? Eating to put on weight gives a feeling of protection, and some degree of reassurance, but feeling full and the actual process of eating sort of adds a bit more to that sense of reassurance. Does that sound right?'

Julia thought about it. 'It feels good to eat, that's the bottom line, and whilst, yes, I can say it feels good to be able to wear this jacket, to feel that I've made healthy choices, it doesn't *feel* the same, it's not such a sharp experience as, yes, a new word, the sense of relief that comes with eating, and eating to feel full. Yes, there is that satisfaction, but there's also a sense of relief, of feeling right in some way. It doesn't feel right not to be eating.'

'OK, something about a sense of the relief that comes from eating and also a sense of rightness, that it feels right to eat, to feel full?'

'That feels more like it. And that rightness, yes, that includes protection, reassurance, relief, everything. Yes, it's what feels right.'

'Mhmm, it feels quite simply right to eat in a particular way.'

'Not even in a particular way, just right to eat.'

'OK, I've got that, it quite simply feels right to eat, and to not eat, or to change your eating habits . . .'

'Simply does not feel right, however much I know the logic of it, inside it just doesn't feel right.'

Pamela nodded, feeling sharp and focused and feeling a genuine intensity in the dialogue once again. It felt like a genuine exploration, trying to get hold of what was happening for Julia and finding words to capture it.

Sometimes it can really feel as if you are working together to find the right words to get a joint grasp of an experience, a sensation, a feeling, an emotion. Gradually the words are refined, the client feels she is more accurately understanding herself and that the counsellor also has an understanding of what she is experiencing. She has been able to identify a sense of how right it feels to eat, that it is something quite fundamental to her eating experience. And the dialogue continues with a further insight into where she carries the sense of rightness in herself.

'Yes, it doesn't feel right to not eat the way that you are used to eating and, bottom line, want to continue eating.'

Julia opened her mouth to agree, and hesitated. 'And . . ., and I know it's not right. In my head I know it's not right. But it feels right.'

'Mhmm, in your head it's clearly right to change, but that rightness hasn't reached your feelings. The rightness in your feelings is about carrying on eating as you have been.'

'Yes, yes, it's like the change hasn't really hit my feelings, not really. I thought it had, but it hasn't. I've changed my behaviour and I've made myself begin to think differently, but my emotions are stuck, lagging behind.'

'Stuck . . .?'

Julia smiled, 'In the past.'

Pamela nodded.

They both lapsed into silence. It felt as though an important point had been reached. For Julia it felt important for her to have found that insight. It was as if she really *knew* something. She could see it, feel it. For Pamela there was a sense of reaching a fresh vantage point, that the dialogue in the session with all its intensity had brought Julia to this point. What would happen next, she had no idea. It would be trustworthy, though, whatever it was. Julia would make of what she had just said, what she had realised for herself, and the process of getting there, whatever she would.

Julia was shaking her head. 'I feel strangely calm again, but it's a different calm. It's like, well, it's like it's OK. It's like I can see it, understand it in some way. I can't really put it into words, but I can see that, yes, my feelings are stuck in the past. It makes sense. I make sense. It wasn't making sense before. It just felt like . . . , I think I used the word "craziness".'

'You did. And yes, you see yourself differently, see things as they are.'

Julia was aware of suddenly feeling very tired. She felt quite drained and felt a yawn coming on. She raised her hand to her mouth. 'Oh, sorry, I suddenly feel really tired.'

'I'm not surprised, you've done a lot of work this session, and experienced a lot of emotion as well.'

'I feel like I need time to think about all of this. I think I want to go and sit in the park.' She had glanced out of the window and saw that the sun was shining, 'just sit and be, look at the flowers. Yes, just be a little bit at peace with myself.'

'Sounds a great place to be. Enjoy it.' Pamela smiled. The session ended and Julia left, heading for the park, walking slowly, thoughtfully, and yet purposefully, a woman who wasn't sure quite where she was heading in life, but who seemed to have at least a clearer sense of what she had to leave behind.

Pamela was also feeling quite drained. She had been concentrating so hard in the session, particularly towards the end, no, she'd been concentrating throughout but that last dialogue had really been intense, trying to be sure she was hearing and understanding Julia, and putting back what she was sharing in a way to help Julia feel heard and able to explore her feelings further.

Points for discussion

- How has the session left you feeling?
- How has the session left you thinking?
- Evaluate the effectiveness of Pamela's therapeutic responses.
- What enabled Julia to reach her own truth about herself?
- What is your reaction to thinking in terms of 'parts', and to the notion that we can find ourselves suddenly dominated by parts of ourselves rooted in past experiences?
- Discuss the session in terms of the working of person-centred theory and Rogers' seven stages of change.
- Write notes for this session.

CHAPTER 11

An overview

Something changed in that last session for Julia. It was as though she was seeing the reality, no, more than seeing, she had experienced the reality of the split inside herself. The following few sessions continued with reviews of her changed eating pattern, her occasional release of further emotion linked to her past and her fears associated with her weight change, and a gradual emergence of a woman with increasing self-confidence. She continued to lose weight and explored ways of healing the split between the part of herself that was so strongly linked to the sexual abuse, and the person she was seeking to become. She realised that it was not a case of it being a battle or a fight, that what she needed to do was to find ways of healing the differences within herself, of finding ways for a reconciliation.

Pamela continued to offer a therapeutic climate based on the presence of the necessary and sufficient conditions for constructive personality change. Greater openness developed between them; Julia finding it easier to express her feelings, to be open to what emerged for her through the process of counselling and her changing eating pattern. She felt more accepting of herself. She could really and genuinely appreciate what had happened to her, psychologically and mentally, she could make sense of herself. She was less afraid of the part of her that wanted her to eat, and slowly, that part also began to lose its fear of what would happen when Julia's weight reduced.

This process of change occurred slowly, with Pamela being attentive to all that Julia said, offering a safe and supportive environment for the fears from whichever part of Julia to be heard and warmly accepted. Julia began to recognise signs and symptoms within herself when the urge to binge eat to put weight back on emerged, although it was less and less about putting weight on as simply seeking the satisfaction from the eating experience and from feeling full that brought that sense of reassurance that she had highlighted earlier.

Her emotions began to mature, as well, as though they were now beginning to play 'catch-up'. Julia found herself going back to the music she had heard as a young teenager. She began to trust her feelings, allow them to be more present. She began to encounter feelings for men, feelings that at first were strange to her, that she had previously kept at bay and simply refused to feel, losing herself

153

in the eating experience. Now, well, now she was beginning to accept that those feelings were OK. She was questioning what she had taken from her experience as a young teenager, the things that the boys next door had said to her. She allowed herself to begin to make her own judgements, tentatively at first, about the men around her – mainly those at work. She rejected, more and more, what she had carried with her for so long, and the anxieties began to diminish, the urge to eat in the old ways faded.

Julia continued with the counselling, changing it to fortnightly and beginning to shift the tone of the sessions in a way that left Pamela feeling she was a kind of, not exactly a mother figure, Julia didn't need that, she was having a good relationship with her mother; more of a confidant, a trusted friend, with a certain 15 or 16 year old tone to it. Pamela appreciated that this was part of the process and valued her time with Julia, journeying with her as she encountered new feelings and talked about new experiences that were coming her way.

It is now three months later and Julia has lost more weight, the jacket she so proudly wore is now too large and has been consigned to the back of the wardrobe as a reminder. She spends less time now talking about eating in the sessions, that has become less of an issue. Yes, she did have eating binges during those three months, but they were explored and made sense of, and generally Julia was able to contain them herself. She learned from them. Since session 18 she had been more able to observe herself, get to know who she was in a way that was different to before. She brought more self-awareness into her life, and the way she made sense of things was less dominated by her thoughts and feelings from the past.

Having a place where she could be herself, could feel safe to express herself, was so important to her. It was like a place she could let go of things, explore things, talk about anything she felt she needed to make sense of. She found it fascinating.

Her course had begun at work and she was doing well with that, and it meant she had met new people on the course. She had begun to talk about one young man who she felt drawn to, but she had kept her distance. She found it difficult talking about him in the counselling sessions without getting embarrassed. These were feelings and experiences that were in so many ways new to her. It is now session 27.

Counselling session 27: exploring reactions to a date and a relationship

'He asked me out.' Julia felt all excited and a little bit coy as she told Pamela. 'Well, I mean, I just, well, I didn't know what to say. I felt myself colour up, I know he noticed, he told me later. I just said "oh", can you believe it. My tongue felt like it was three times its usual size. I thought, "be cool". Cool!'

'So, you got a lot of reactions, then, and found it hard to speak.' Pamela was aware that she was smiling. There was such a wonderful freshness now about

Julia, and she really appreciated it. She guessed it was Mark from her accountancy course, she'd been talking about him and had said how they had exchanged a few words a few times, but nothing more.

'I was like a teenager. I know we've talked about that and I've recognised it but this was like, I mean, it was something else. So, anyway, I managed to string a few more words together. Know what I said? Oh God. No, I didn't say that, I said "that would be nice". Can you believe it? "Nice". Yuk. How did I say that? I'm surprised he didn't run away. But he didn't and, well, we went for a drink and then to the cinema. The film was OK, well, actually I don't remember much of the film. I mean, well, I was *so* self-conscious. What am I like? I was so aware of him there, next to me. Oh God. And he was so relaxed and we really, really enjoyed it. It was about Peter Sellars. We decided to go to it as we both wanted a bit of a laugh. I thought I was messed up! No, that's not fair, but he was in some ways a bit like me, Peter Sellars, that is – as though something hadn't quite grown up. I mean, everything else is different, but there was something that made me think. I guess people have all kinds of problems and difficulties, and find the best way they can to deal with them. He lost himself in different characters, in playing roles even in his relationships. At least, that's how it seemed. I lost myself through eating.' Julia paused.

'Something strike you?'

'Just the way I said it, that I lost myself through eating. That's true, isn't it, I mean, I did lose myself, at least I lost the possibility of growing and developing in the way that I might have done if things had been different, if that bastard William hadn't got to me.'

'Mhmm, lost yourself through eating because of William.'

Julia could reconnect with her experiences now without the same emotional upset, if anything it was now more a case of feeling anger. As she had questioned what she had been told, as she had begun to accept that it was a horrible thing that he/they had done, then the main emotion was anger towards him/them.

'Who knows how I would have been.' She thought for a moment. 'Life could have been very different, who knows. But I wouldn't have probably been doing what I am doing today. Probably would have been married, I suppose. You don't know, do you?'

'No, the only reality we know for certain is the one that we have. Everything else is a series of "what ifs". You may have been married, or stayed single and travelled, maybe had a whole series of boyfriends.'

Julia pulled a face. 'Now I think you're teasing me.'

Pamela smiled, and shrugged her shoulders with a very clear false look of innocence.

The relationship is firmly established. This kind of lightness has its place – it is about people being normal, expressing themselves, bringing a humorous touch to the therapeutic experience. It would not be appropriate early

> on when a relationship is establishing itself, and a client needs to experience their counsellor as trustworthy and accepting. Humour can confuse clients who are sensitive and vulnerable in relationship.

'OK, well, maybe, but, well, I have what I have and for now I'm going out with Mark.' Julia looked very pleased with herself.

'It's serious, then?'

'I don't know about that, but maybe it is. I feel good being with him, you know, I've never felt like that before.'

Pamela was aware of feeling pleased for Julia and also concerned as to how vulnerable she might be. She maintained her empathy. 'A new experience, it feels good being with him.'

'I feel sort of freed up, somehow, it's hard to explain. We discovered we like the same kinds of music, and we've been out twice more, and had numerous phone calls. My head's in a spin.'

'I'm really pleased, it sounds wonderful. You really are having a lot of contact.'

'Yes. But . . .'

'But?'

Julia took a deep breath and sighed. 'Well, I mean, there are two things really. I mean, I'm sort of worried, I mean, given what happened to me in the past, how will I react to us getting, you know, closer. I mean, we've kissed but, well, I don't know how I'm going to feel, how I'll react if he wants sex.'

'If he wants sex?'

'I guess it's not just him, is it, it'll be me as well. I mean, it's just that, oh I feel quite silly.' Julia looked down. She was suddenly feeling quite flustered.

'Mhmm, what'll happen when he, or both of you want to become more physical with each other.'

'I mean, I haven't . . .'

'And it's worrying you.'

Julia nodded. 'Teenagers do it all the time today, and here am I, 26, getting all anxious.'

'And it's right to honour that anxiety. It's a big step for you.'

Julia nodded. 'I suppose it is, and more so than for others. And, I mean, well, I know I've lost weight, but I'm still big and, well, I mean, will he be turned off? Oh God, this feels awful. I mean, I've thought about it, of course I have, and worried about it. And I just feel so nervous, and I really don't feel very confident. But when I'm with Mark somehow I'm not thinking or feeling like this. It's afterwards, when I have time to think and, well, yeah, that's the problem.'

Pamela was aware that Julia had said that there were a couple of things, but she decided not to remind her, maybe she had captured the second issue in what she had said. She didn't want to take her focus away from what had emerged.

'So it feels good when you are with him, but afterwards when you think about getting more intimate, then you get nervous.'

'I guess I have to just go with it. I just want it to be OK.'

'Yes, yes, it's important for you to feel that it will be OK.'

'Do people worry like this? I suppose they do, but not quite like this. I mean, oh I
don't know.'

'It's confusing, and hard to know if others feel like you?'

'I guess so. I mean I do like him a lot. So I suppose, yes, I am thinking that one day
we'll have sex together.'

Pamela noted a reaction in herself around Julia's use of language. She wondered,
will they have sex, or will they make love? Or both? She, herself, was clear that
there could be a very definite distinction.

'Mhmm, one day you'll have sex together.'

'I guess it'll happen when it happens?'

'Mhmm, let it happen naturally as an expression of what you feel.' Pamela knew
she was slipping into giving advice but it somehow felt right to have said it.

Maybe it is right for Pamela to say what she has said, in the context of the
feelings that Julia has for Mark. But sex doesn't have to be an expression of
love, it can be a release, it can be an exploration, it can be about dominance
and being dominated, it can mean an income, it can be so many different
things for different people. Who knows what it will mean for Julia? She has
to discover her own meanings and the counsellor should keep her meanings
outside of the counselling room.

'I suppose, in a way, it is like that first kiss, only more so.'

'And you've come through that experience.'

Julia nodded. 'And that just felt so easy, so right, so good, so sweet ... Listen to
me! Sorry, I was drifting off then.'

'You really do care deeply about him?'

Julia took a deep breath and nodded. 'Hopeless case, fall in love with the first man
that asks me out.'

'That how it feels, that you're a hopeless case because of falling in love?'

'Probably not, but I do a bit.' Julia paused, remembering the last evening that
they had been together, and she was seeing him again that night, they were
going out for a meal. Oh, yes, she remembered, that was what she wanted to
talk about as well. 'The other thing is that, well, we're going out for a meal
tonight, to an Indian restaurant and, well, I know in the past I always ordered
too much and ate too much. I didn't think that then, of course, but now looking
back I know I did. And I guess we'll go out for meals at other times and, well, I
need to make sure I don't let myself go. I mean, I'm already noticing an urge to
eat when I feel good, and as I'm feeling good a lot of the time, well, that definitely isn't good.'

'So, feeling good has become an eating trigger.'

'I don't think it's become, maybe it was always there, but it's more present at the
moment. And I really need to watch it.'

'So, I feel good, so I'll eat to ...' Pamela looked at Julia as she wasn't sure how to
finish what she had said.

'... to feel even better. It's crazy, but it's like I feel good and so I'll just eat something and ...' She paused and smiled. 'Ah.'

'Ah?'

'You remember I talked about how things felt right when I was eating, when I eat
a certain amount?'

'Mhmm.'

'Well, maybe that's it. I feel right when I have eaten, and somehow it gives the
good feelings an added sense of rightness.'

'That feels really perceptive, that the food adds a slightly different quality to the
experience of feeling good, gives you a sense of rightness in some way.'

Julia nodded, 'and I have to watch that. I really do. I don't want to go and start
putting weight on now'.

They discussed what she might eat, given that most Indian restaurants seemed to
offer similar menus, something that Pamela had always found frustrating, and
since she had been diagnosed with high blood pressure she had avoided them
because she was concerned about the level of salt – the food always tasted so
salty. She realised that was true in lots of other restaurants as well. She pulled
her thoughts back to Julia who was now deciding what she would have.

'So, I'll have one poppadom to start, and I'll keep away from the fried rice, and
have plain boiled rice, that's OK. And I guess I need to keep away from anything
too creamy or fatty, so maybe a straight curry would be best. And one side dish.
Maybe the chick peas, chana masalla, isn't it, or the spinach, that's the sag
aloo. Yes, but only one. And no naan bread, that can be quite oily as well, and
really fills me and I don't want to get back into eating to make myself feel really
full. I've learned not to do that. You know, one of the hardest things I've
learned these last few months is that it is OK to leave food on your plate. That
just seemed so foreign to me. Breaking the habit of eating because it's there and
developing an eating habit because I feel hungry – and I mean hungry, not
bored, or as something to do whilst watching TV.' She shook her head. 'I've
learned a lot, haven't I?'

'Yes, and pretty much self-taught. You've worked things out for yourself, made
choices, tried different strategies, found what works and built on it.' Pamela
wanted to ensure that Julia acknowledged how much was down to her.

'I couldn't have done it without you. I know you made a few suggestions – trying
to make me eat ice-cream with a smaller spoon, I recall!'

'That's a bit overstated, don't you think?'

'No, but I can't say I blame you.' Julia stopped to reflect. 'A lot of change, and
more change on the horizon. My life, my horizon, are expanding.'

'And I'm so pleased, so many new possibilities opening up for you.'

'And I'm in a place in myself now where I can begin to take them. I've decided I'm
going to cook one of the meals we learned at the cookery class for Mark.
Haven't quite decided which one, but that will be quite a big thing.'

Pamela wondered how soon, whether Julia would want to talk about it, but she
wasn't going to ask her. She trusted Julia to know what she needed to bring to
these sessions. They were, after all, her client's time.

The session moved on to bringing Pamela up-to-date about Julia's relationship with her mother. She was beginning to feel that she wanted to say something to her about what happened with Jake and William. She was beginning to experience a sense that somehow it would be right to share it with her, not to blame, but to help her mother perhaps make sense of how she, Julia had been, and why she was changing. She had told her about the counselling, but only that it was about helping her to reduce her weight and change the way she ate. She hadn't made up her mind what to say or when, but it felt good airing it with Pamela. She realised that somehow it was important for her to feel that her mother understood her, and she left the session a little more certain that she would, at some point, tell her. But not yet. Her thoughts moved on to getting herself ready for the meal that evening. What to wear? Yes, life felt a lot better, she felt a lot better. She knew she still had to watch herself, and that maybe she always would, there were always tempting reasons to slip back into old patterns of thought and feeling that would encourage her eating pattern to change back to how it had been. So, maybe she was ten years behind the clock, but she was feeling good and she was, after all, a 26 year old, going on 16, with a hot date on her mind. Her pace quickened as she headed home to get ready. Yes, she was feeling a bit anxious, of course she was, but she was also smiling. And she wasn't aware that she was no longer looking down at the pavement as she walked.

Reflections

Pamela's reflections – 'It's so good to see Julia freeing herself up and moving on in her life. She could so easily have been held back even longer by her experience of sexual abuse. It's not just the physical act, the words used, the images of what she could expect in the future were, in their own way, as abusive, perhaps some might argue more so, but that's a debate for others to have. It did stifle her growth, and now she is catching up. I pray that she will not feel drawn to someone who will, in any way, treat her in such a way that the old fears are rekindled.

'As for the counselling process, yes, it wasn't easy at times to resist offering advice, and I know that at times I did just that. But I tried to ensure that I felt connected and any thoughts that I voiced were ones that had emerged during times of close connection with Julia. I don't want that to sound like an excuse, I think there are times for a person-centred counsellor to share a view, but not in such a way as to undermine the client's developing internal locus of evaluation.

'Something did happen in the session when Julia realised for herself, and in her own way, that her emotions were stuck in the past. There was something about that session. For me it felt that I was most true to being person-centred in some way, staying with Julia, maintaining and communicating my empathy as she explored herself, trying to find the right words, and me then trying to find the right words to convey what I had heard – so difficult to do and avoid falling in the trap of merely saying the words that the client has said. Empathy is so much more than that. In fact, in many ways the verbal empathy may be secondary to the primary empathy which is the actual attention and listening, the attitude that enables the client to feel listened to and heard at the time they are speaking. And I was holding and experiencing my feelings of warmth and unconditional positive regard for her as well. It is exhausting to be that focused, and energising in a strange way. There is something nourishing for the counsellor when he or she is able to connect deeply with a client. It's not just the client who gains, there are two people in the room and in a way the counsellor changes as well as a result of the relationships they form with clients. Funny that, because they're not receiving empathy from the client. Hopefully the client is becoming more congruent, but how much unconditional positive regard they hold towards the counsellor, well, that varies I'm sure. And yet it does encourage change.

'So, I am optimistic for Julia. Yes, there will no doubt be difficult patches but I hope that the psychological and emotional changes she has been through, and is going through, will ensure that her outer behavioural changes around her eating will be sustained. I think they will be. I think Julia has a very different relationship now with herself. That may sound strange, but her 'intra-relationships' have evolved significantly, and they are more satisfying to her, and she is engaging in lifestyle changes that are bringing further satisfying experiences. She is now evidencing greater unconditional positive self-regard. What greater encouragement can there be than your own personal experience of feeling more accurately self-aware and that in line with a greater self-awareness there is a strong sense of "rightness" about the choices you are making in your life.'

Julia's reflections – 'I've been asked to comment on the counselling that I've experienced. Phew! What can I say? When I started to attend well, it felt OK, a chance to talk a few things over, which I did, and my mood lifted. But then, well, then I had to start to talk about my weight and my eating, that was something I really didn't want to do. It was only because of what had been said at work that I knew I had to do something. And I tried doing it myself but, well, I seemed to end up eating more. And then, once I'd started to talk about it I knew where I was heading, and I didn't want that, I hoped it would go away, wouldn't have to be talked about. But it did, and it was. And I felt better for it, though at the time I'd rather have been anywhere than sitting in that room.

'Pamela listened, she really did listen. And that was important to me. Having someone there. It was good that she made a few suggestions at times as well, but that wasn't the important thing. I just needed someone to let me be me, I guess, let me say what I needed to say in the way I needed to say it.

'I feel so fortunate to have met Pamela. I'd seen her leaflet and when things got on top of me I happened across it again at home, and, well, gave her a call. I like the way she tries to understand me, and that was particularly important when

I was really trying to make sense of what was happening to me, and how I was so still caught up in ways of thinking and feeling that were rooted in my early teenage years.

'I know I still have some way to go, but I think I'm now able to grow not only within the therapy sessions, but outside as well. As I was thinking about what to say, that came to mind. At first, well, the only place that I felt any different was with my counsellor. Nothing was changing at home or at work, life was almost on hold in a way, just doing what I had to do, but there was no sort of, I don't know, spark I guess like there is now. Now I feel like I'm growing, learning, developing in all areas of my life. I suppose that's what therapy is supposed to do, give you a boost, fire you up. Well, I guess it's more about offering something to enable me to fire myself up, I'm sure Pamela would remind me that I've done most of the work. I can accept that, but I needed that other person, and she was that other person, someone who I could pour things out to, struggle with myself with, feel accepted for who I am – and who I am becoming. Yes, I think Pamela would like it said that way. It certainly feels right to me.

'So, my life moves on. I shall continue to see Pamela for a while; I really want to get myself how I want to be. I'm still learning, still finding things out. And I'm sure that being with Mark is going to bring even more things out. I am anxious about it, but I guess that's normal. I'd like to feel more confident and in a way I am when I am with him, but when I am back home on my own, the doubts creep in, the worries, the uncertainties, all the "what ifs".

'Anyway, I feel like I have given myself a chance now of a very different future, and I must grasp it. Whatever happens, it has to be better than living with feelings that had got themselves stuck in a horrible period of my life. Those two years – they affected me badly for over ten years now, and I don't want them messing up the next ten, or the ten after that. I'm grateful for the chance to be different and life, for the moment anyway, and hopefully it will continue, feels good, and what I am doing feels right, and that's so important.'

Points for discussion

- What are your thoughts and feelings about Pamela, about Julia, and about the way that the person-centred approach has been portrayed?
- How do you sense Julia to have changed at this, the end of session 27, and how would you relate this to Rogers' seven stages of change?
- Taking the whole counselling process, what were the key themes for Julia and how effective was Pamela in responding in a person-centred manner?
- If Julia was to relapse on her changed eating pattern, what would you anticipate could be the likely causes? How would you need to respond if you were her counsellor?
- Write notes for this session.

Author's epilogue

It is strange writing these books. The characters get under your skin, their journeys whilst fictitious, take on a certain reality. Not everyone, of course, will have the experiences of Steve and Julia. Everyone with a problem related to over-eating will have their own unique reasons, experiences, and ways of responding to a need to lose weight. Not everyone will have underlying emotional issues to deal with, but many will, and they may not be aware of them at first. And not everyone's obesity, as mentioned at the start of the book, is due solely to over-eating, although most overweight problems are directly as a result of over-eating – too many calories with not enough expenditure of energy. Only about 1 per cent of obesity cases are medication- or endocrine-related.

I always have mixed feelings at this stage – I feel pleased to have finished writing the book, and particularly so with this one. What I have read about the damaging effects of obesity has made me aware of how this issue needs to be responded to, and I felt strongly that I wanted to describe the role of person-centred practice in this situation. My feelings are mixed, though, because I always want to extend the stories further, look ahead, find out what happened next in the clients' lives. Does Steve get to sixteen stone? What else changes in his life? Does he get over his health problems? And Julia. Her new relationship, how will it develop? Will she find a satisfying relational experience? How will her life turn out? Of course, I know they are fictitious, and yet, sometimes they can begin to feel quite real. As I say, they get under your skin.

Whilst this book, like all the books in the *Living Therapy* series, is written to give the reader an experience, to bring them in touch with a client, or clients, and their particular set of difficulties and challenges, there are also the counsellors to consider. What of John and Pamela? How has their work, as it has been portrayed, impacted on you? What have you learned from their mistakes, and from those successful moments when movement occurs, those creative moments when it is as though time stands still as a client grasps something or sees something for the first time, or in a new light, or those painful struggles that the counsellor witnesses and is affected by as some deep-seated pain and hurt bursts into awareness and into the therapeutic space?

The supervisors, too, offer another set of material to reflect on and to be affected by. Is there anything from them which has stayed with you? Would they be supervisors you would consult and, if so, why, and equally, if not, why not?

Sustainable change

I feel strongly that there is a need to recognise that for behaviour change to be sustained, there is a need for emotional and psychological change. And with an increasing focus on obesity issues within the context of healthcare, this recognition must be taken fully into account when working with clients. Otherwise, yes, a person may change their eating pattern, and may lose weight, but do they really free themselves from the emotions and thoughts that are linked to their eating, or their size? People may change outwardly but still live in a perpetual nightmare of struggle within themselves. For instance, like Julia, who if she had not begun to address the emotional issues from her past and how it affected her, would be likely to be left in a constant battle with herself, possibly entering a cycle of binges and inner stress and as a result maybe doing herself more harm than good.

Whatever the particular cause of a person's obesity, the simple fact remains that a person is more than the shape of their body. We all have feelings and thoughts, habits, fears, joys, hopes, memories, sadnesses; and have similar needs, to be loved, respected, listened to, valued. It may seem an obvious thing to say but in the critical and condemnatory language that is spoken towards and about people who have an obese or an overweight condition, it can get forgotten.

Defining the problem

Whilst obesity is clearly a physical health problem, I would argue that it is *not* necessarily a mental health problem. Yes, there are mental health components and for some people their obesity will be linked to binge-eating, body dismorphia, and may have associated anxiety and depressive states. Some obese people will be mentally unwell, and that will be linked to their obese condition – as cause and/or effect. But obesity *per se* is a symptomatic effect of causes that can be wide-ranging and complex: psychological and physiological, with societal, familial and economic factors contributing to the condition. For many people, as with some other mental disorders, they have simply developed a way of coping with their experience of life. Once we associate obesity with mental illness I believe we are on dangerous ground. Each person must be considered as an individual. Simply because someone behaves in a way that is damaging to their health is not a basis for a mental health diagnosis. Yes, some people will be obese and will have a concurrent mental illness that may be diagnosable in line with current mental health diagnostic parameters; but not everyone.

If anything, it is perhaps society that has the illness. Obesity is a symptom of this illness. Dominant food producers have sought to profit from high-energy foods and consumers have been seduced into the fashionable image of processed foods and the prevailing value that more is better. Obesity is more prevalent in lower social class groups. Without doubt, if the trends towards increased levels of obesity are to be reversed, it will require a political will that places the health and well-being of citizens above the profit margins of food producers. And that will require a major shift in values in societies where the producers control the market and the advertisers shape the demand. Somehow, somewhere, somebody has to start taking responsibility – producer, advertiser and consumer – along with governments who, it would seem, have for too long favoured the interests of the producers and those at the business end at the expense of the health and well-being of the consumers. Obesity is perhaps a symptom of a far deeper social ill, the culture of 'big is better'. Sometimes it is, but not always.

We also have to look at lifestyles as well. We live more sedentary lives. Transport systems mean we indulge less in walking, and one-stop shopping in vast supermarkets or shopping malls means we have no need to walk large distances. More and more work seems sedentary as people sit at desks viewing computer screens. There is a need for discipline to get up, take a walk, burn a bit of energy. Lifestyle changes need to be promoted as well as changes in diet.

The person-centred response

The person-centred approach to counselling people with obesity issues honours the many facets of their personhood. It offers a disciplined approach, applying a tried and tested theory in creating the therapeutic conditions and experiences that can promote the constructive personality change that Rogers describes. As a result the client will become more authentic in their personhood. This, in turn, encourages changes to the behaviours that they had developed out of being the person that they were. These changes will ensure that their behaviours in the present more accurately reflect and satisfy the person that they are in process of becoming. In this process they can be trusted to address the obesity issue to the degree that they are able and motivated so to do, reflective of the changes within their personality or structure of self. They will move at their own pace. And the changes that are made, because they result from changes within the very structure and nature of their personhood, will be more likely to be sustained. In the final analysis, successful change is sustainable change.

Of course, not everyone will view successful change as meaning the same thing. For some people it may mean a loss of weight, but for someone else it might mean change to a healthier diet, a more positive body image, increased self-confidence, a raising of self-esteem, a better overall sense of weight management, a liberation from thoughts and feelings about themselves that were rooted in conditional experiencing in the past. And there will be those people who decide not to make major changes, or for whatever reason feel it is impossible. For them, small changes in diet and lifestyle to minimise the impact of their over-eating may be viewed as a successful outcome.

With obesity still on the increase we are all likely to find ourselves working with clients who are either overweight or who are obese. I hope this book has raised awareness of issues related to obesity, and to the role of the person-centred counsellor. I also hope it has demonstrated the importance of the relational experience for the person seeking to change an eating pattern that is linked to psychological and emotional factors. I hope that it will have left you, the reader, with much to ponder on for your own practice.

Appendix 1

Rogers' seven stages of constructive personality change[1]

Stage 1
'There is an unwillingness to communicate self. Communication is only about externals.

Feelings and personal meaning are neither recognized nor owned.

Personal constructs are extremely rigid.

Close and communicative relationships are construed as dangerous.

No problems are recognized or perceived at this stage.

There is no desire to change.

There is much blockage to internal communication.'

Stage 2
'Expression begins to flow in regard to non-self topics.

Problems are perceived as external to self.

There is no sense of personal responsibility in problems.

Feelings are described as unowned, or sometimes as past objects.

Feelings may be exhibited, but are not recognized as such, or owned.

Experiencing is bound by the structure of the past.

Personal constructs are rigid, and unrecognized as being constructs, but are thought of as facts.

Differentiation of personal meanings and feelings is very limited and global.

Contradictions may be expressed, but with little recognition of them as contradictions.'

Stage 3
'There is a freer flow of expression about the self as an object.

There is also expression about self-related experiences as objects.

---

[1] Extract from *On Becoming a Person* (1967) by Carl Rogers, pp. 132–55. Reprinted by permission of PFD on behalf of Carl Rogers. © Carl Rogers 1967.

There is also expression about the self as a reflected object, existing primarily in others.

There is much expression about or description of feelings and personal meanings not now present.

There is very little acceptance of feelings. For the most part feelings are revealed as something shameful, bad, or abnormal, or unacceptable in other ways.

Feelings are exhibited, and then sometimes recognized as feelings.

Experiencing is described as in the past, or as somewhat remote from self.

Personal constructs are rigid, but may be recognized as constructs, not external facts.

Differentiation of feelings and meanings is slightly sharper, less global, than in previous stages.

There is a recognition of contradictions in experience.

Personal choices are often seen as ineffective.'

Stage 4

'The client describes more intense feelings of the "not-now-present" variety.

Feelings are described as objects in the present.

Occasionally feelings are expressed in the present, sometimes breaking through almost against the client's wishes.

There is a tendency towards experiencing feelings in the immediate present, and there is distrust and fear of this possibility.

There is little open acceptance of feelings, though some acceptance is exhibited.

Experiencing is less bound by the structure of the past, is less remote, and may occasionally occur with little postponement.

There is a loosening of the way experience is construed. There are some discoveries of personal constructs; there is the definite recognition of these as constructs; and there is a beginning questioning of their validity.

There is an increasing differentiation of feelings, constructs, personal meanings, with some tendency toward seeking exactness of symbolization.

There is a realization of concern about contradictions and incongruences between experience and self.

There are feelings of self responsibility in problems, though such feelings vacillate.'

Stage 5

'Feelings are expressed freely in the present.

Feelings are very close to being fully experienced. They "bubble up", "seep through", in spite of the fear and distrust which the client feels at experiencing them with fullness and immediacy.

There is a beginning tendency to realize that experiencing a feeling involves a direct referent.

There is a surprise and fright, rarely pleasure, at the feelings which "bubble through".

There is an increasing ownership of self feelings, and a desire to be these, to be the "real me".

Experiencing is loosened, no longer remote, and frequently occurs with little postponement.

The ways in which experience is construed are much loosened. There are many fresh discoveries of personal constructs as constructs, and a critical examination and questioning of these.

There is a strong and evident tendency towards exactness in differentiation of feelings and meanings.

There is an increasingly clear facing of contradictions and incongruences in experience.

There is an increasing quality of acceptance or self-responsibility for the problems being faced, and a concern as to how he has contributed. There are increasingly freer dialogues within the self, an improvement in and reduced blockage of internal communication.'

Stage 6

'A feeling which has previously been "stuck", has been inhibited in its process quality, is experienced with immediacy now.

A feeling flows to its full results.

A present feeling is directly experienced with immediacy and richness.

This immediacy of experiencing, and the feeling which constitutes its content, are accepted. This is something which is, not something to be denied, feared, struggled against.

There is a quality of living subjectively in the experience, not feeling about it.

Self as an object tends to disappear.

Experiencing, at this stage, takes on a real process quality.

Another characteristic of this stage of process is the physiological loosening which accompanies it.

The incongruence between experiences and awareness is vividly experienced as it disappears into congruence.

The relevant personal construct is dissolved in this experiencing moment, and the client feels cut loose from his previously stabilized framework.

The moment of full experiencing becomes a clear and definite referent.

Differentiation of experiencing is sharp and basic.

In this stage, there are no longer "problems", external or internal. The client is living, subjectively, a phase of his problem. It is not an object.'

Stage 7

'New feelings are experienced with immediacy and richness of detail, both in the therapeutic relationship and outside.

The experiencing of such feelings is used as a clear referent.

There is a growing and continuing sense of acceptant ownership of these changing feelings, a basic trust in his own process.

Experiencing has lost almost completely its structure-bound aspects and becomes process experiencing that is, the situation is experienced and interpreted in its newness, not as the past.

The self becomes increasingly simply the subjective and reflexive awareness of experiencing. The self is much less frequently a perceived object, and much more frequently something confidently felt in process.

Personal constructs are tentatively reformulated, to be validated against further experience, but even then, to be held loosely.

Internal communication is clear, with feelings and symbols well matched, and fresh terms for new feelings.

There is the experiencing of effective choice and new ways of being.'

Appendix 2

'Cycle of change' model

Another way of approaching change is to take a more cognitive-behavioural perspective and to focus specifically on the behaviour that is being changed and the attitude of the person towards that behaviour. The 'cycle of change' model, devised in the early 1980s by two American psychologists Prochaska and DiClemente (1982) describes the process and stages people pass through when undergoing change in terms of behaviour and attitude towards that behaviour, and ways of working to encourage them to change. It was originally devised in relation to smoking, but has been widely applied to working with people who have addictive behaviours for instance, in relation to drug and alcohol use. Recently, one of its co-authors has produced his own book (DiClemente, 2003), offering a more detailed description of the application of this model in treating addiction. It is an approach that has also been applied to working with patients having weight problems (Sharman, 2004). The 'cycle of change' model suggests that people pass through stages each of which has certain characteristics and demands particular areas of focus and response in order to help the client move on. The stages are:

- pre-contemplation
- contemplation
- preparation
- action
- maintenance
- lapse or relapse.

Pre-contemplation

In this stage the client will not be thinking about change. This may because they simply do not see their weight as a problem or as something needing to be addressed. It could be that they do recognise that it has become an issue, but find the idea of change too difficult or uncomfortable to consider and have pushed the idea aside. This might be described as 'denial'; although it is worth acknowledging that this stage is not necessarily a negative one. Being in denial when someone is aware that there is a problem which they are uncomfortable about and seeking to push the discomfort aside, means that the client is in a state of incongruence. This, as we have seen, is one of the necessary conditions for constructive personality change. If the person-centred counsellor can offer warm and genuine acceptance of the client's need to deny the difficulty, and can empathise with that behaviour and the resulting discomfort, change may happen. Often the pushing away of a problem is a psychological reflex, and when it is explored within a supportive therapeutic climate, it can be broken down and/or re-evaluated, with the possibility of a different outcome.

Contemplation

At this stage the client is more in touch with, and accepting of their discomfort about, in this context, their eating and weight, and is entering into a process of thinking about change, exploring it and what it would mean. This can be a lengthy process. People can, and do, take time to make decisions that involve change, particularly those that affect them directly and intimately. Weight, body size and shape and eating habits contribute to a person's identity and sense of self. They will not necessarily be changed easily and quickly, and may involve a good deal of exploration and heart-searching. The process cannot be hurried. The client needs time to genuinely consider the pros and cons of change, and to really understand, for themselves, what they might be embarking upon and why.

It is that stage at which a client may be keeping a diary of their eating to understand the quantity, pattern and type of food being eaten. Also, the triggers for eating may be identified. It is a time for the person to really get as full an understanding of their eating pattern and the meanings that they attach to their eating pattern as possible. The latter is important and can get overlooked where there is a rush made towards behaviour change. Food can mean many things to different people, and particular foods may have particular meaning, for instance, certain foods may be comforters, whilst other foods may be eaten more when the client is in a particular mood, or with particular people. All of this is important to recognise so that the client can be as fully informed as possible as they consider their options. This information embraces both the client as a person and the eating pattern itself.

During contemplation a client may decide, for whatever reason, not to pursue change. They will have reasons for this, and these must also be warmly and genuinely accepted. Sometimes, as a result of this acceptance, the client may revisit the process and change their mind, others will not. They may break from the counselling, or may wish to stay in the counselling relationship perhaps to work on another issue. At least if the client chooses not to change, it is possible that their perspective on the problem will have changed and, given different circumstances at a future point, they may draw on this to make changes.

Preparation

The contemplation stage is also helping the client to inform themselves in readiness for the stage of preparation. At this point the client will have recognised that, yes, on balance, they want to make changes and begin to plan their strategy. They will formulate their goals and it is important that they are owned by the client, and are realistic. Too many people lapse because goals are unrealistic, having been set more from the agenda of the counsellor than the client. They also need to have a clear time-frame to work within, again which must be owned by the client and be realistic. In terms of an eating pattern, this could involve reducing or cutting out particular foods or drinks, reducing portions and cutting out or reducing 'snacking'.

Unlike with alcohol, you cannot seek abstinence from food. But you can seek abstinence from certain foods. In effect, for the person seeking to resolve eating issues and a weight problem, their process is more about achieving a 'controlled eating' regime. Also, there will perhaps be an element of 'harm minimisation'. This is a useful term which would mean cutting out or cutting down on food and drink that is particularly damaging to health, or foods that are likely to cause weight gain.

Risks of lapse or relapse are also discussed, and ways of minimising them, or of responding to them, planned. It is better to have ideas formulated in order to avoid a slip in the controlled eating regimen, rather than have to try and find a solution afterwards. A person will feel good about achieving an avoidance of a lapse, and this can be built on to enhance motivation.

Action

Having created the strategy for change it then has to be put into action. Quite simply, this is the stage at which the plan is enacted. Support systems will now be in place as well as systems to enable the client to self-monitor. The client may continue to keep a diary of their eating pattern, and of their weight. However, whilst weight loss may be an eventual aim, this can become a barrier to achieving a change in the eating pattern. Yes, it can be a motivating factor, but if weight is not lost, it can sap motivation. For some people, simply focusing on a more healthy diet, or a reduction in quantity without too much emphasis on weight can be helpful. Sometimes, the early stages of change simply require the breaking up of the pattern that is established, helping the person to begin to appreciate that they have choices, that they can decide to eat something else. Eating patterns can become habitual – we eat today what we ate yesterday, because we ate it the day before. Eating can go on to a kind of 'automatic pilot'. The shopping is only done at certain shops. Certain foods are bought because of familiarity. Encouraging a sense of adventure can be helpful, for changing an eating pattern is an opportunity to experience something new. It is not always solely about giving something up.

Maintenance

Change must be maintained, but for how long before it is deemed a sustainable change? It will vary from person to person, and depends largely on their psychological responses to opportunities or triggers to return to the original eating pattern. Monitoring should continue and high-risk situations be thought through. It may take some time before the person feels that they are no longer having to make themselves avoid eating something, or maintain portion control. The person has to pass through a psychological process of accepting themselves as a person who doesn't eat a particular foodstuff, or doesn't have to eat everything on their plate, or can actually feel good about taking time to eat a smaller portion for the taste rather than eating for the experience of quantity.

Lapse or relapse

There may be slips, blips, when more is eaten, or chocolate biscuits creep back into the eating pattern. These can be usefully explored. There will be a reason why, and it is likely to be associated with a feeling or an experience. It may be something identified during contemplation/preparation, but for which the planning has not proved adequate. Or it may be something unexpected, which requires a process of exploration leading to informed planning as to how to deal with it should it arise again. There may be an underlying emotional issue to work through.

The task, at this stage, is to ensure that a lapse does not become a relapse. This will have been discussed in the preparation phase. Also, to ensure that the client does not break contact so that they can be encouraged to continue with their effort, if they wish to, learning from what has occurred. It can be depressing to lapse, and tempting to give up. Change is not easy and counsellors must appreciate this. The temptation to eat is all around us. It is a fact that problem drinkers have difficulties watching television programmes that are so centred in pubs, or where alcohol is being consumed regularly. For the person who is struggling with an eating issue, imagine how it would be if TV programmes were constantly centred in cake shops, or cafés frying food all the time. At least the drinker can try and avoid the off-licence, the pub, or the alcohol displays in the supermarkets, but you can't avoid places where there is food on display.

Exit from stages

As we have seen, there are exit points from the cycle. Clients may exit the process either in contemplation or preparation if they feel that the time is not right for change, or simply find themselves unable to sustain their motivation. They may exit the cycle from maintenance having achieved their goal, whether that is a change of eating habit and/or achieving and maintaining a certain level of weight loss. Finally, they may exit from lapse or relapse, going back into their previous pattern of eating as a result of which they may choose not to try to change, or they may return to pre-contemplation to weigh up and learn from their process so far.

What is key is to bear in mind that whilst there is change taking place in eating behaviour, this has to be underpinned by a psychological process of change. The person-centred counsellor does not direct the client around the model, it exists to inform the process. Clients often find it interesting to have a handout so they can think, for themselves, what the different stages mean to them. They may see different stages, or want to use their own language to define their process. All of this is perfectly reasonable and acceptable. But the psychological process of change must not be lost sight of in the rush to achieve behaviour modification. Gradual and informed change, sustained over time, is more valuable than a cycle of constant failure which can be psychologically debilitating and undermine the person.

Appendix 3

Controlling what is eaten

In her book *Counselling for Eating Disorders*, Sara Gilbert makes reference to over-eating, and includes some interesting and helpful cognitive-behavioural techniques and perspectives, along with information about binge-eating, attitudes to fat, stress-induced eating and relapse prevention (Gilbert, 2000). She identifies six areas that are important to be recognised and applied where someone is seeking to change an eating pattern in which they eat when they see food, when they see other people eating, or when they are thinking about food.

1 Eat only in one place.
2 Do nothing else while eating.
3 Eat only with a knife and fork.
4 Make eating extra snacks and helpings more difficult.
5 Shop with a list.
6 Avoid extreme hunger or boredom.

By applying these, the person dissociates eating from everywhere and rather learns to associate it with a particular place or environment. It helps people to avoid the temptation to carry food from room to room. It also leads in to the value of making eating a particular and specific experience, and not something to accompany or be associated with other activities. 'I always watch TV when I eat,' can easily then become 'I always eat when I watch TV'.

Eating only with a knife and fork can slow down the eating process, but it can also make it difficult to eat certain foods, particularly snacks. It has a restrictive effect. Added to this, if a conscious effort not to bring snack foods into the home is made, smaller portions are cooked, smaller plates are used which look fuller and perhaps more appealing than a reduced helping on a large plate, then further restrictions are established. Also, if snacks have to be in the home, maybe they should be stored in a particularly inaccessible cupboard. Leftovers are also another source for snacking. Prepare and/or cook only what is required, and perhaps, though some might feel it is wasteful, throw away any surplus (Gilbert, 2000, pp. 152–4).

176

Gilbert also emphasises the need for people to consider whether their urge to eat is genuine hunger, or for some other reason from which they may be able to distract themselves. Also, if they are fast eaters, can they slow down, for instance, putting the knife and fork down between mouthfuls, deliberately chewing food more, perhaps also to dwell more on, and therefore maximise, the flavour experience.

There is also the choice of where people shop. The health food shop may be an accessible alternative. It may be more expensive, but the person reducing their food intake will be saving by buying less. It is an environment in which there should be less temptation to buy high fat, high calorific and simply unhealthy food and drink. If a person has to go to the supermarket, try to develop 'speed shopping', or 'shopping with a purpose'. By bringing an attitude into the experience of not wanting to hang around in the supermarket any longer than necessary, temptation can be minimised. A client might even want to take pride in reducing the time they take shopping, going in for what they want and then getting out. There is more to life than spending time in supermarkets.

References

Adams P (1993) *Gesundheit*. Healing Arts Press, Vermont.

Banegas JR, Lopez-Garcia E, Gutierrez-Fisac JL *et al.* (2003) A simple estimate of mortality attributable to excess weight in the European Union. *European Journal of Clinical Nutrition*. **57**: 201–8.

Bentall RP (1990) The syndromes and symptoms of psychosis. In: RP Bentall (ed.) *Reconstructing Scizophrenia*. Routledge, London.

Bozarth J (1998) *Person-Centred Therapy: a revolutionary paradigm*. PCCS Books, Ross-on-Wye.

Bozarth J (2002) Empirically supported treatments: epitome of the specificity myth. In: JC Watson, RN Goldman and MS Warner (eds) *Client-centred and Experiential Psychotherapy in the 21st Century: advances in theory, research and practice*. PCCS Books, Ross-on-Wye, pp. 168–81.

Bozarth J and Wilkins P (eds) (2001) *Rogers' Therapeutic Conditions: evolution, theory and practice*. Volume 3: *Unconditional Positive Regard*. PCCS Books, Ross-on-Wye.

Bryant-Jefferies R (2001) *Counselling the Person Beyond the Alcohol Problem*. Jessica Kingsley Publishers, London.

Bryant-Jefferies R (2003a) *Counselling a Recovering Drug User: a person-centred dialogue*. Radcliffe Medical Press, Oxford.

Bryant-Jefferies R (2003b) *Time Limited Therapy in Primary Care: a person-centred dialogue*. Radcliffe Medical Press, Oxford.

Bryant-Jefferies R (2003c) *Counselling a Survivor of Child Sexual Abuse: a person-centred dialogue*. Radcliffe Medical Press, Oxford.

Department of Health (2004) *Health Survey for England 2003*. DOH, London.

DiClemente CC (2003) *Addiction and Change*. The Guilford Press, New York.

DiClemente CC and Prochaska JO (1998) Towards a comprehensive, transtheoretical model of change: stages of change and addictive behaviours. In: W Miller and N Heather (eds) *Treating Addictive Behaviours* (2e). Plenum Press, New York.

Embleton Tudor L, Keemar K, Tudor K *et al.* (2004) *The Person-Centered Approach: a contemporary introduction*. Palgrave MacMillan, Basingstoke.

Evans R (1975) *Carl Rogers: the man and his ideas*. Dutton and Co., New York.

Gaylin N (2001) *Family, Self and Psychotherapy: a person-centred perspective*. PCCS Books, Ross-on-Wye.

Gilbert S (2000) *Counselling for Eating Disorders*. Sage, London.

Hallam RS (1983) Agoraphobia: deconstructing a clinical syndrome. *Bulletin of the British Psychological Society*. **36**: 337–40.

Hallam RS (1989) Classification and research into panic. In: R Baker and M McFadyen (eds) *Panic Disorder*. Wiley, Chichester.

Hallett R (1990) Melancholia and Depression. A brief history and analysis of contemporary confusions. Unpublished Masters Thesis, University of East London.

Haugh S and Merry T (eds) (2001) *Rogers' Therapeutic Conditions: evolution, theory and practice*. Volume 2: *Empathy*. PCCS Books, Ross-on-Wye.

House of Commons (2004) *Health Committee's Report on Obesity*. HMSO, London.

Kirschenbaum H (2005) Carl Rogers' life and work: an assessment on the 100th anniversary of his birth. *Journal of Counseling and Development*.

Kutchins H and Kirk S (1997) *Making us Crazy: DSM: the psychiatric bible and the creation of mental disorders*. The Free Press/Simon Schuster, New York.

Mearns D and Thorne B (1988) *Person-Centred Counselling in Action*. Sage, London.

Mearns D and Thorne B (1999) *Person-Centred Counselling in Action* (2e). Sage, London.

Mearns D and Thorne B (2000) *Person-Centred Therapy Today*. Sage, London.

Merry T (2001) Congruence and the supervision of client-centred therapists. In: G Wyatt (ed.) *Rogers' Therapeutic Conditions: evolution, theory and practice*. Volume 1: *Congruence*. PCCS Books, Ross-on-Wye, pp. 174–83.

Merry T (2002) *Learning and Being in Person-Centred Counselling* (2e). PCCS Books, Ross-on-Wye.

National Audit Office (2001) *Tackling Obesity in England*. National Audit Office, London.

Patterson CH (2000) *Understanding Psychotherapy: fifty years of client-centred theory and practice*. PCCS Books, Ross-on-Wye.

Prochaska JO and DiClemente (1982) Transtheoretical therapy: towards a more integrative model of change. *Psychotherapy: Theory, Research and Practice*. **19**: 276–88.

Rogers CR (1942) *Counselling and Psychotherapy: newer concepts in practice*. Houghton-Mifflin Company, Boston, MA.

Rogers CR (1946) Significant aspects of client-centered therapy. *American Psychologist*. **1**: 415–22.

Rogers CR (1951) *Client Centred Therapy*. Constable, London.

Rogers CR (1957) The necessary and sufficient conditions of therapeutic personality change. *Journal of Consulting Psychology*. **21**: 95–103.

Rogers CR (1959) A theory of therapy, personality and interpersonal relationships as developed in the client-centred framework. In: S Koch (ed.) *Psychology: a study of a science*. Volume 3: *Formulations of the person and the social context*. McGraw-Hill, New York, pp. 185–246.

Rogers CR (1967) *On Becoming a Person*. Constable, London. (Originally published in 1961.)

Rogers CR (1980) *A Way of Being*. Houghton-Mifflin Company, Boston, MA.

Rogers CR (1986) A client-centered/person-centered approach to therapy. In: I Kutash and A Wolfe (eds) *Psychotherapists' Casebook*. Jossey Bass, San Francisco, pp. 236–57.

Sharman K (2004) From compliance to concordance: a psychological approach to weight management. *Healthcare Counselling and Psychotherapy Journal*. **4** (4). BACP, Rugby.

Slade PD and Cooper R (1979) Some difficulties with the term 'schizophrenia': an alternative model. *British Journal of Social and Clinical Psychology*. **18**: 309–17.

Thorne B (1996) Person-centred therapy. In: W Dryden (ed.) *Handbook of Individual Therapy*. Sage, London.

Tudor K and Worrall M (2004) *Freedom to Practise: person-centred approaches to supervision*. PCCS Books, Ross-on-Wye.

Vincent S (2005) *Being Empathic: a companion for counsellors and therapists*. Radcliffe Publishing, Oxford.

Warner M (2000) Person-centred psychotherapy: one nation, many tribes. *The Person-Centred Journal*. **7**(1): 28–39.

Warner M (2002) Psychological contact, meaningful process and human nature. In: G Wyatt and P Sanders (eds) *Rogers' Therapeutic Conditions: evolution, theory and practice*. Volume 4: *Contact and Perception*. PCCS Books, Ross-on-Wye, pp. 76–95.

Weiner M (1989) Psychopathology reconsidered. Depression interpreted as psychosocial interactions. *Clinical Psychology Review*. **9**: 295–321.

Wilkins P (2003) *Person-Centred Therapy in Focus*. Sage, London.

Wyatt G (ed.) (2001) *Rogers' Therapeutic Conditions: evolution, theory and practice*. Volume 1: *Congruence*. PCCS Books, Ross-on-Wye.

Wyatt G and Sanders P (eds) (2002) *Rogers' Therapeutic Conditions: evolution, theory and practice*. Volume 4: *Contact and Perception*. PCCS Books, Ross-on-Wye.

Useful contacts

Person-centred

Association for the Development of the Person-Centered Approach (ADPCA)
Email: adpca-web@signs.portents.com
Website: www.adpca.org

An international association, with members in 27 countries, for those interested in the development of client-centred therapy and the person-centred approach.

British Association for the Person-Centred Approach (BAPCA)
Bm-BAPCA
London WC1N 3XX
Tel: 01989 770948
Email: info@bapca.org.uk
Website: www.bapca.org.uk

National association promoting the person-centred approach. Publishes a regular newsletter *Person-to-Person*.

Person-Centred Therapy Scotland
Tel: 0870 7650871
Email: info@pctscotland.co.uk
Website: www.pctscotland.co.uk

An association of person-centred therapists in Scotland which offers training and networking opportunities to members, with the aim of fostering high standards of professional practice.

World Association for Person-Centered and Experiential Psychotherapy and Counselling
Email: secretariat@pce-world.org
Website: www.pce-world.org

The Association aims to provide a worldwide forum for those professionals in science and practice who are committed to, and embody in their work, the theoretical principles of the person-centred approach first postulated by Carl Rogers. The Association publishes *Person-Centred and Experiential Psychotherapies*, an international journal which, 'creates a dialogue among different parts of the person-centred/experiential therapy tradition, supporting, informing and challenging academics and practitioners with the aim of the development of these approaches in a broad professional, scientific and political context'.

Obesity and eating issues

National Obesity Forum
PO Box 6625
Nottingham NG2 5PA
Tel: 0115 8462109
Website: www.nationalobesityforum.org.uk

Overeaters Anonymous
PO Box 19
Stretford
Manchester M32 9EB
Tel: 07000 784985
Email: info@oa.org
Website: www.oagb.org.uk

The British Dietetic Association
For practical advice about healthy eating visit its consumer website.
Website: www.bdaweightwise.com

The Obesity Awareness & Solutions Trust (TOAST)
Latton Bush Centre
Southern Way
Harlow CM18 7BL
Tel: 01279 866010
Email: enquiries@toast-uk.org.uk
Website: www.toast-uk.org.uk

Index

T - #0662 - 101024 - C0 - 246/174/11 - PB - 9781857757286 - Gloss Lamination